Acknowledgements

I am profoundly grateful, beyond measure, to my wife, Barbara, whose love and incredible patience has shown that every day our marriage gets sweeter and more profoundly phenomenal. Indeed, not only is she my wife of over 43 years, she is the mother of our two wonderful sons Andrew and Christopher, but she is also my compass. Barbara is my lover and my friend. As a very qualified professional, educator, and professional speaker, she is also my attorney and my counselor. She has kept the Smith family, and all the endeavors of the various Smith businesses, on course throughout our wonderful journeys.

D1399093

Other Books by Thomas A. Smith

Aromatherapy: a Primer for Health Professionals

The Essential Guide to Essential Oils

To Barbara

First Printing: June 2014	Sixty-third Printing: December 2017

ISBN-13: 978-1499295665
ISBN-10: 1499295669

For information on this and other books, seminars, trainings, consulting services, etc. please contact Smith Rehabilitation Consultants, Inc. at:

http://www.mentalhealthseminars.net

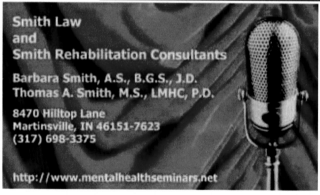

The material presented in this book is for educational purposes only and should not replace the advice or treatment plan of a physician or other health care practitioner. It should not be used for diagnostic or prescribing purposes. The author offers no endorsement of products, recommendations for drug dosing, or implied promises of relief. Case studies, references, charts, and images used throughout the book are for illustrative purposes only and should not be used as models for medication management of any particular disorder. Every attempt was made to present accurate information at the time of publication, but the subject of psychopharmacology is an ever-expanding one. The author assumes no responsibility or liability for any action take as a result of the information contained in this book.

Psychopharmacology Made Simple:
A Primer

First, do no harm...

Table of Contents:

Where does one "find" mental illness in the body?

In the field of medicine, some PET scans and CAT scans are used in the "diagnosis" of mental illness, as well as some magnetic imaging studies (fMRI). The quandary is "where is mental illness located?"

Can this question be definitely answered? Well, science is not completely sure!

There will be some detailed history in a few pages, but for now, consider:

Yes, Galen said that the brain controlled the rest of the body, and Descartes, St. Thomas Aquinas, and philosophers and physicians and mystics and laity and the learned have argued about that subject: "Where is mental illness found?" for centuries and centuries.

To look at the answers, consider this ethical question-
Have you, gentle reader, ever "seen" depression on a PET scan?
- Or have you "seen" increased electrical activity in a section of a brain, or increased glucose metabolism, or spirit activity, or organic response to outside stimuli, or...
- Can you "see" ADHD?
- SPECT analysis has been used to try to answer this question. Understand that some of the available SPECT research has been peer reviewed- some not.

What do the initials **"SPECT"** represent?
Single **P**hoton **E**mission **C**omputerized **T**omography.
What about the **initials "PET"**?
Positron **E**mission **T**omography.

So what is being represented by these "scans?" Photons? Positrons? Are these truly "showing" ADHD, depression, etc.? For a fascinating- and current- review of this controversy, the reader is directed to an article by Anderson et al:

Our findings point toward a fundamental tension between academic investigators on the one hand, and commercial service providers on the other. This scenario poses dangers to the communities directly involved, and to public trust in science and medicine more generally. Much work needs to be done to mitigate these dangers and maximize the potential of exciting new technology. With a focus on the patient and the collective strengths of both the research and service provider communities, constructive steps can be successfully understand to achieve these parallel goals. (Anderson, Mizgalewicz, & Illes, 2013)

The controversy continues... in *The New Phrenology-The Limits of Localizing Cognitive Processes in the Brain,* written by William R. Uttal.

Dr. Uttal questions the use of imaging, and: "...is concerned that in an effort to prove itself a hard science, psychology may have thrown away one of its most important methodological tools--a critical analysis of the fundamental assumptions that underlie day-to-day empirical research." (Uttal, 2003) In his book Uttal addresses the question of localization: specifically, whether psychological processes can be defined and isolated in a way that permits those processes to be associated with particular brain regions.

More from Dr. Uttal:

"New, noninvasive imaging technologies allow us to observe the brain while it is actively engaged in mental activities."

"Uttal cautions, however, that the excitement of these new research tools can lead to a neuroreductionist wild goose chase. With more and more cognitive neuroscientific data forthcoming, it becomes critical to question their limitations as well as their potential." (The MIT Press, 2003)

Uttal reviews the history of localization theory, presents the difficulties of defining cognitive processes, and examines the conceptual and technical difficulties that should make us cautious about falling victim to what may be a "neo-phrenological" fad. Oh, incidentally, William R. Uttal is Professor Emeritus in the Department of Psychology at the University of Michigan and in the Department of Industrial Engineering at Arizona State University.

Understand that there are branches of science that may be considered "hard science"- such as:

<u>Physics</u>   <u>Mathematics</u>   <u>Chemistry</u>   <u>Astronomy</u>

And other branches that are not as "hard":

<u>Pharmacology</u>   <u>Medicine</u>

As well as some branches that might be considered "soft" sciences...

<u>Psychology</u>   <u>Philosophy</u>

<u>Goodness, indeed the goal of science is to try to be scientific!</u>

But how hard is it to get volunteers to be the control cohort on a suicide or ECT study?

Note also that this topic, psychopharmacology encompasses scientific theories from all the above branches.

As an example, regarding "science":

Scientists link month of birth to diseases

Adapted from *The Indianapolis Star,* August 20, 2004:

"Pisces (February 19 – March 20):
Governed by Neptune and symbolized by the fish.
Compassionate, introspective, artistic.
Often dreamy and impractical.

> May be prone to schizophrenia, epilepsy, or bipolar disorder!" (Lallanilla, 2004; Niedowski, 2004).

Even narcolepsy- a condition with diagnostic specifics found in the *DSM-5* (American Psychiatric Association, 2013) - has been related to "the month of birth." Per Dr. Emmanuel Mignot, professor of psychiatry and behavioral sciences at Stanford University School of Medicine, as published in the September 2003 edition of the journal *Sleep* (Dauvilliers, Carlander, Molinari, Desautels, Okum, Tafti, Montplaisir, Mignot, & Billiard, 2003), corroborated by published research in Britain and Norway. Mental illness and "birth month" correlations have also been affirmed by Dr. E. Fuller Torrey, research psychiatrist at the Uniformed Services University of Health Sciences in Bethesda, MD. (Davies, Welham, Chant, Torrey, & McGrath, 2003) The astrological implications of mental illness have been addressed by Professor McMahon at Vanderbilt. (Ciarleglio, Axley, Strauss, Gamble, & McMahon, 2011)

Environmental factors are very difficult to study and are very speculative, says Dr. Emmanuel Mignot, professor of psychiatry at Stanford University, whose research discovered the increase in narcolepsy among people born in March. It's nearly impossible to find out what could be involved, like finding a needle in a haystack. (Foster & Kreitzman, 2010)

Remember, the goal is to try to make psychology a "hard science"
And this is done for:

Professional identity	*Results that can be replicated*
Reimbursement	*To try to help our patients*
Research funding	

It is time to address some basic concepts...

Just what are "drugs?"

This simple question has many answers-
Beginning...

First, one may say that "drugs" are chemicals that the body uses to produce a desired therapeutic result, either in a single organ; or, an entire system. Or, one might say that drugs are substances which replace the normal physiological functions and/or psychological functions that are either:

℞ Absent from the body; or,

℞ Present in the body in insufficient concentrations to produce the desired effects.

Or, one might say that drugs are substances which mimic a normal physiological or psychological presentation.

Or one might say that drugs are chemicals that alter the way that the body works...and each of the above would be right on all counts!

As an example, insulin is used to replace low insulin levels, patients will take calcium supplements to replace bone loss, and clients take caffeine to keep awake.

Clients take laxatives to facilitate "normal bowel function."

✹ Hey, what do these have to do with the subject today?
Good question!

The correlation between these seemingly disparate topics is that drugs (or, for that matter, psychotherapies) are used to modify "normal" functioning.

Note that different "types" of drugs (and again, therapies) may be used to achieve the same desired outcome.

The overriding concern in these statements is that we have no clue as to what exactly IS "normal?"

When talking about drugs used in psychotherapy, we are talking about drugs that may affect:

Mood   **Personality**   **Behavior**
So, are:
Mood   **Personality**   **Behavior...**
...able to be quantified as "normal?"

Is "normal"...

Socially acceptable?	Ethnically based?
Functionally defined?	Assessed by third-party standards (government, educational, testing, etc.)?

After finishing this book, the hope is to have these and many other questions addressed...

✹ But probably not answered completely...

However, there is a part of this book that may provide some answers-

✹ The part dealing with psychopharmacology

History is rich with information regarding drugs and therapies...

For example, trepanning is from the prehistory-the drilling of holes into the skull to relieve "illnesses" like headaches, hallucinations or visions, hearing voices in the head.

The Egyptians not only developed mummification, but also the concept of "taking a history" from the patient. The Egyptians also found out about herbal medicines through their trading links with other countries.

In the time of King Solomon, the Iron Age IIA (1000 to 900 B.C.E.) one finds the advent of other "chemicals"-

* Specifically aromatherapy. (Smith, 2013)
* Sandalwood was all throughout King Solomon's Temple; sandalwood is a natural antiseptic. Indeed, one might say that when a person went into King Solomon's Temple that he or she was "cleansed" and left "feeling better." Sandalwood to this day is used in the Far East to make funeral boxes.

The Greeks and Romans continued with herb therapies...

Galen, the "Father of Pharmacy" (he was in reality a physician), first suggested that the brain was in "charge" of the rest of the body.

The Greek Physician Scribonious Largus in the year 47 A.D. came up with 241 "prescriptions" at the request of the Emperor Claudius's freedman Gaius Julius Callistus. One of these therapies was to put electric eels on the heads of patients cure headaches.

During the Middle Ages...

There were several outbreaks of bubonic plague, called "the Black Death". People tried many different ways to prevent and cure the Black Death. There were herbal medicines, superstitious remedies, recipes for clearing the air of "miasma," and religious punishments.

None of these remedies worked, because people did not actually understand what caused the plague.

There were some improvements in medicines, as a result of the many wars in this era, which in turn led to an increase in the number of doctors, and these doctors began to use wine as an antiseptic to treat wounds.

These doctors also used opium as an anæsthetic.

Only men were allowed to be doctors; if women practiced medicine they were hanged as witches.

The Renaissance ushered in...

Explorers who traveled to far off lands, bringing back plants which were used as medicines, one was the bark of a tree, the cinchona tree, which contained quinine, used to treat malaria. Another plant was tobacco.

Physicians and scientists also began understanding the human body better, as autopsies were now "allowed." William Harvey explained the circulation of blood throughout the body in 1628.

The 18th and 19th centuries brought about...

Nitrous oxide and chloroform, Edward Jenner, Louis Pasteur, Florence Nightingale, and Robert Koch.
> ➤ Ah! And the discovery of microscopic "things!"

History also includes the use of homeopathy and aromatherapy...

For example, the use of *Lycopodium Clavatum*, also known as Club Moss, Wolf's Foot, Staghorn, and Vegetable Sulphur. This was used by "ancient physicians" as a stomachic and diuretic. *L. Clavatum* was described as a "polychrest with antipsoric, antisyphlitic, and antisychotic properties."[1] (Weiner & Goss, 1989)

The "mental" part of L. Clavatum:

The Lycopodium patient may appear extroverted, capable, but with a peculiar detachment, a sense of his own superiority. With the slightest suggestion of illness, he becomes hypochondriacal, headstrong, and haughty. Averse to company, yet dreads solitude; wants someone in the adjacent room.

Sadness and gloom, better moving about a while.
Psychosomatic ailments, particularly gastrointestinal (Weiner).

The 20th century...

Began with penicillin, blood transfusions, vaccines, and insulin, and ended with radiography, gene therapy, and DNA studies.

And the 21st century includes...

Pharmacogenomics and psychoproteins, or drugs that work for individual patients, with several pharmaceutical companies on the forefront of this technology, for example:

Genaissance Pharmaceuticals, Inc., Valda, Eli Lilly, and Roche Diagnostics.

---

[1] In this reference, the words "polychrest", "antipsoric", and "antisychotic" are not misspelled- this is a direct quote from the reference.

Great! So you, gentle reader, have now had a (very) short (and truncated) history of medicine.

But here's one of the more difficult- and truly fascinating- aspects of this book:

From where did the drugs currently used to treat mental illness come?

The answer may be a surprise- most of these have a basis in...infections!

Indeed, most clinicians just know that these medications exist, and have had the different types of drugs drilled into the minds of those clinicians as a result of college, seminars, and clinical practice.

But what was the driver that caused these medications to "be"?

Note that while there has been a history listed in this book, **THE DIRTY LITTLE SECRET HAS BEEN- AND IS-** that medications are given to people with mental illnesses. If the medications "work" then those medications are given to other patients with similar symptoms.

Reflect back on the concept of "penicillin" above. Indeed, this was one of the significant sources of mental health treatment- infections. Patients were sick (with infections.) Penicillin often cured the infection. In short, people got sick, penicillin made those people feel better.

But hold on, here! Can one consider any current mental health clinical presentations that are caused by infection?

Upper respiratory infections (especially in the elderly clients, often in residential care) may appear to have dementia-like symptoms. Clear up the infection, clear up the mental health presentation.[2]
Urinary tract infections (again, more often encountered in the elderly patient, but UTI and URI can cause symptoms in any age patient) which also may appear as mental confusion, irritability, depression, and a host of other symptoms typically diagnosed as being in the realm of mental illness.
Late tertiary syphilis (the patient is asymptomatic for the syphilis lesion) which may also be misdiagnosed as being dementia.
Meningitis may have different clinical presentations; for example, newborns may appear to be "fussy", sleep quite a bit more than expected, and be irritable. Older patients may complain of headaches, seizures, decreased appetite, being photosensitive, and difficulty in awakening.[3]
PANDAS- the acronym stands for: **P**ediatric **A**utoimmune **N**europsychiatric **D**isorders **A**ssociated with **S**treptococcal Infections. This syndrome appears after a child has had a streptococcus infection (strep throat; Scarlet Fever) and may have a dramatic, overnight onset. Symptoms? PANDAS may look like Tourette Syndrome, and the children who develop PANDAS may have Obsessive Compulsive Disorder symptoms. Of note is that the OCD as a rule does not respond to the typical psychotherapy or pharmacotherapy interventions currently used to treat OCD. PANDAS occurs between age 3 and puberty. Sometimes PANDAS may be mistaken for ADHD, separation anxiety, sleep disturbance, night-time bedwetting (and frequent urination during the day), mood changes (including irritability, sadness, and emotional lability[4]), and even joint pain.

So, indeed, infection may be significantly intertwined with mental illnesses.

---

[2] Interesting, this is often called "silent pneumonia." The patient showing the mental confusion may not have a fever- may not even have difficulty in breathing. But upon viewing a chest x-ray, is often found to have a fulminant pneumonia.

[3] Viral meningitis (often called "aseptic meningitis") and bacterial meningitis have the same clinical presentation- but the bacterial meningitis is much more severe and needs medical attention immediately. Viral meningitis usually resolves successfully in most patients who have a functional immune system.

[4] Here is something to consider- often the "clinical presentation" of depression is children is linked to an increase in "irritability."

That is where psychopharmacology has been focused- penicillin is a "magic bullet." Take penicillin and it really does not matter "where" the infection may reside, the drug "kills" the bug[5]. The goal has been- and still is- to find the "mental health magic bullet." (Whitaker, 2010)

Now, look at another significant infection, and see how this plays not only into this book but also psychopharmacology.

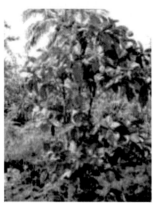

Royalty *Cinchona pubescens,* a species of *cinchona*, taken by CH Lamoureux (University of Hawaii). (Reproduced by courtesy of Prof. Gerald D Carr, Department of Botany at the same University). (Kaufman & Rúveda, 2004)

Malaria kills millions of people worldwide. There has been a very effective treatment of malaria- quinine[6]. Quinine may be obtained from the cinchona plant (mentioned in the preceding section of this book dealing with the "quick medical history.)

The problem is that there are millions of people who contract malaria, and there are not enough plants to supply the quinine to fulfill that demand.

So, medicine (and society) turned to the chemists with this question:

"Can you make synthetic quinine?"

The answer is, "Yes!"

And, by the way, this is not a difficult synthesis.

Understand, though, that one does not just "start" with a raw material and WHAM! arrives at the intended medication. Chemists have to go through several steps of synthesis to arrive at the goal.

Chemists are an intriguing lot. Not only do the chemists look at developing a specific chemical entity, but the chemists also look at the intermediary products that occur as a result of following those specific synthesis steps. In the chemistry world (and pharmacology world) some significant discoveries have occurred by accident. Serendipity was the mainstream source of results.

Starting with petroleum, a rich source of carbon (remember that humans are carbonaceous creatures) one may perform several chemical reactions, and come upon various other chemicals that have some pretty interesting properties.

---

[5] Obviously, penicillin does not "kill" all bacteria. This is used for analogy only, and one could make an argument that Prozac doesn't "cure" every depression.

[6] Malaria had become resistant to quinine, so the pharmacologists, chemists, and pharmacy manufactures developed several "super quinine" derivatives. Malaria has been very busy, and is now resistant to many of these "super quinine" medications. There is evidence that quinine once again may be used to treat malaria.

As an example, in developing quinine to treat malaria, chemists used petroleum as the starting raw material. Petroleum contains aniline chemical compounds. By chemically messing with one of those aniline compounds, one can arrive at a chemical most persons reading this book will find as being a part of his or her personal history. Reflect back to high school biology. Remember the first time looking through a microscope at a human cell? Remember the wonderful world one found there? Now, remember that one might use a "stain" to change the cell so that various parts of the cell would be more visible. Shucks, if one got some of that stain on one's skin, it might turn the skin purplish blue.

That bluish stain was known as methylene blue, and is made from aniline:

Methylene blue obviously changes cells (it stains cells, and gives them color and definition.) Hey, wait! Maybe one could give methylene blue to patients who have cells that are not working well? Like...patients with mental illnesses!

Methylene blue worked for those patients with mental illnesses! **Not well**. But it did help some patients. It is still used for many conditions, including "memory enhancement." Of interest, methylene blue is a monoamine oxidase inhibitor, so it could theoretically be used to treat depression and Parkinson's disease. Some more information on methylene blue is that this chemical is still used internally in medicine today for various conditions, and that the use of methylene blue has been known to be associated with serotonin syndrome (US FDA, 2011)!

Oh, and back to the subject of "mental health drugs having a relationship with infections" understand that the monoamine oxidase inhibitors were originally used to treat "white death" or tuberculosis! (Lieberman, 2003) Indeed, it was noted by observant clinicians that those patients with TB who received these medications "...felt better!"

Chemically manipulating the methylene blue molecule gave medicine the class of antipsychotic medications known as phenothiazines, and this class of medications includes (there are others):

Thorazine	Sparine	Vesprin
Prolixin	Compazine	Stelazine
Trilafon		

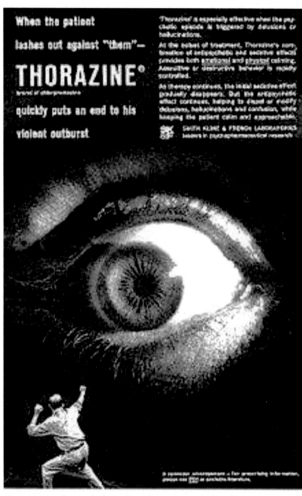

These medications changed society. No longer were mentally ill patients doomed to a life in asylum, but now could be treated in community-based programs. Regarding Thorazine, Edward Shorter wrote, "...imitated a revolution in psychiatry, comparable to the introduction of penicillin in general medicine" (Shorter, 1997).

Oh, and the phenothiazine molecules? Change those molecules a little more and one gets imipramine[7], the first tricyclic antidepressant in the world, known (and still used today) as Tofranil.

The tricyclic antidepressants were thought to "work" on catecholamines in the body, notably, norepinephrine and possibly serotonin. The reason for this theory is again from serendipity, and this will be addressed in the chapter on antidepressants.

All the tricyclic antidepressant medications have a "Daddy" of Thorazine, and a "Great-Great Daddy" of methylene blue. Most of the SSRI antidepressants have some of that "chassis" from methylene blue, and most of the mood stabilizers currently on the market do, too.

---

[7] Methylene blue is closely related to another dye, known as imminodibenzyl- also known as "summer blue" from which many imipramine and other tricyclic antidepressants are derived. Imminodibenzyl is also the "chassis" or "building blocks" for many mood stabilizers, like carbamazepine, discussed later in this book. See Dr. David Healy's wonderful book: *The Creation of Psychopharmacology* (Healy, 2002).

Oh, there is a group of antidepressants that does NOT get the "chassis" from methylene blue...those antidepressants get their DNA (chemical chassis) from a dye that turns skin RED!

One more bit of "history"- here's a really nice chart that describes how psychopharmacology advanced (Depression Hurts. So Do Antidepressants, 2008):

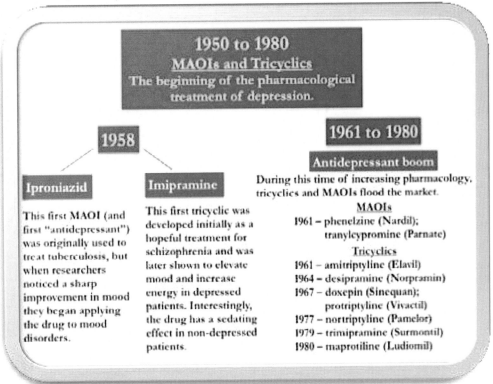

Used with the kind permission of Kate Awsumb, MPH, MA.
(Centers for Disease Control, 2008)

The concept of neurotransmitter activity

Binding sites, agonism, and antagonism

Imagine a nerve cell that releases an electrical nerve impulse after the nucleus is stimulated ("A" below), and that electrical impulse races down the axonal arm, terminating at the axonal buds ("B" below.) Note that there is a "space" between those axonal buds on the nerve cell on the left side of the picture below and the second cell on the right side of the picture. That "space" (right under the "B") is known as the synaptic space or the synaptic cleft.

Those buds at the end of the axonal arm, when stimulated by that electrical impulse, cause a release of neurotransmitters into that synaptic space. The neurotransmitters move across that space and bind with the RECEPTORS found on the dendrites of that second cell (on the right side of the picture below) and then that second cell "turns on."

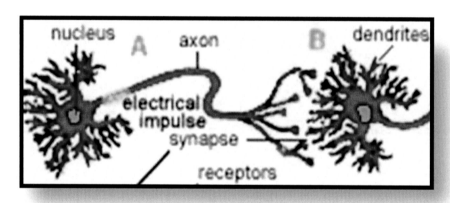

There are two ways an active compound can affect this binding site:

Agonism and antagonism

- Agonists
  - These cause interaction at the binding site to increase the body's normal response.
- Antagonists
  - These compounds cause a "blocking" of the body's normal response.

Binding sites are particular places on the surface of an enzyme or the surface of a cell. When a chemical reacts with an enzyme or a cell, it does so at a binding site. Current theory is that the binding site has a 3-dimensional shape with which a chemical (like a neurotransmitter chemical) interacts with the binding side- rather like a jigsaw puzzle piece fitting into a specific "spot" in the puzzle.

This shape is very important to how that interaction between the neurotransmitter (chemical) and the receptor on the nerve cell "works." The body produces substances (neurotransmitters, specifically) which match binding sites and interact with those binding sites, and this interaction sets off changes in the body.

Finishing "binding sites":

"Diseases," including mental health problems, are thought to occur at a particular binding site. The active compound of a medicine is made to cause something to happen at that particular binding site- either increasing the activity of a specific neurotransmitter, or decreasing the activity of that neurotransmitter.

This is why we have "selective serotonin reuptake inhibitors," for example. SSRIs are thought to work by preventing the "reuptake" of serotonin into the cell that is presynaptic (that is, the cell that is present before the synaptic space, or in the picture above, the axonal buds. When this happen, there is then (theoretically) more serotonin available in the synaptic space.

A graphic example of these concepts:

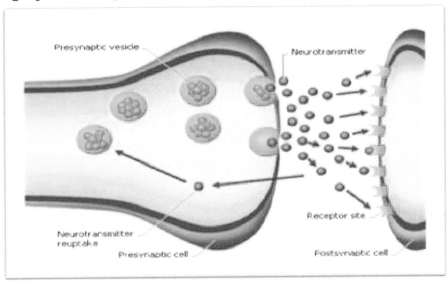

Graphic provided courtesy MindBody Medicine (Peters, 2013.)

17

And now agonism and antagonism (**HOW** the neurotransmitters bind with the receptors):

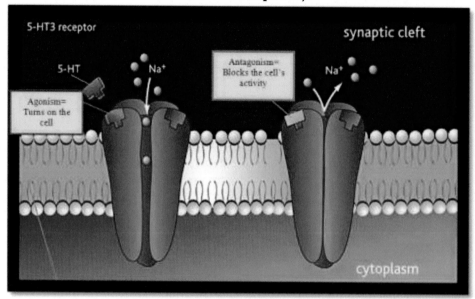

Oh, there is much more to this concept of how the neurotransmitters bind with the receptors. In the Peters graphic above, one can see how the neurotransmitters are thought to migrate across the synaptic space from the presynaptic neuron to the binding sites on the postsynaptic neuron, with some of the neurotransmitters returning to the first nerve cell (the one on the left of the graphic.)

But graphic above, showing the theoretical concepts of agonism (turning the cell on) and antagonism (keeping the cell from turning on.) is often misunderstood. Look carefully at the specific neurotransmitter in the agonism/antagonism graphic where there is the release of neurotransmitter- in this specific case a serotonin molecule- notated at 5HT- that is in the synaptic space and which goes to the binding site on the neuron on the left of that graphic. See how that serotonin molecule "fits" perfectly into that binding site, almost like one would "fit" a jigsaw puzzle piece into a puzzle. The important point of the agonism/antagonism graphic (other than this is how cells are thought to be either turned on or prevented from being turned on) is that the chemical that "fits" is serotonin- 5HT.

There is no such thing as an Abilify receptor in the body; there is no Prozac receptor; there is no Xanax receptor. Nope! There are neurotransmitter receptors, and the current theory is that the medications that people take for mental illnesses are thought to make those neurotransmitters available for binding, or blocking those neurotransmitters from binding.

Why is this big deal? There are thought to be quite a few serotonin receptors in the central nervous system. Here is a list[8]:

- **5HT$_1$**
  - Including 5HT$_{1A}$, 5HT$_{1B}$, 5HT$_{1C}$, 5HT$_{1D}$, 5HT$_{1E}$ and 5HT$_{1F}$
- **5HT$_2$**
  - 5HT$_{2A}$, 5HT$_{2B}$, and 5HT$_{2C}$
- **5HT$_3$**
  - 5HT$_{3A}$, 5HT$_{3B}$
- **5HT$_4$**
  - 5HT$_{4A}$, 5HT$_{4B}$
- **5HT$_5$**
  - 5HT$_{5A}$, 5HT$_{5B}$
- **5HT$_6$**
- **5HT$_7$**
  - 5HT$_{7A}$, 5HT$_{7B}$, 5HT$_{7C}$, and 5HT$_{7D}$

Various serotonin receptors in the central nervous system

Just what does all this mean? It is possible to give a patient radioactive serotonin. Then, a test drug is administered, and a PET scan is taken to see "where the radioactive serotonin accumulates in the brain." Remember this book started with a discussion of PET scans, MRIs, and even phrenology?

If the administration of a specific test medication results in a bunch of radioactive serotonin accumulating in an area of the brain associated with mood, then one could make a statement that "this drug works on mood disorders." If the radioactive serotonin arrived in an area of the brain associated with cognition after the administration of another test medication, then one could make a statement that this second drug "works on dementia."

Indeed, the list of the serotonin receptors above may be broken down into different "areas" of the brain, theoretically:

1. It is thought that mood issues are found in 5HT$_1$;
2. Cognition? 5HT$_2$;
3. Somewhere in 5HT$_3$, 5HT$_4$, and 5HT$_5$ (and oddly, 5HT$_{1D}$) one may find migraine headaches and irritable bowel syndrome.

---

[8] Notice that there is a similarity between the 7 subtypes of serotonin receptors and receptors for dopamine! There are thought to be D$_1$, D$_{2A}$ and D$_{2B}$, D$_3$, D$_4$, D$_5$, D$_6$, and D$_7$ receptors. Parkinson's Disease (remember from the beginning of this book?) is thought to "live" at dopamine D$_1$; psychosis is thought to occur at dopamine D$_2$ receptors.

But once again, there is only ONE dopamine neurotransmitter, and the body will direct the neurotransmitter where the body feels there is a need. This is why one sees Parkinson's medications (dopamine agonists) possibly affecting dopamine D$_2$ receptors as well as the "target" dopamine D$_1$ receptors- resulting in Parkinson's patients wigging out (hypomania, mania, even psychosis) or hypersexuality (pain, PLEASURE, and rage!)

This is also why when dopamine D$_2$ receptors are blocked (antagonists) with antipsychotic medications, that some patients develop "hand tremors" and even gait disturbances that are clinically identical to those encountered in the clinical presentation of patients with Parkinson's Disease. Is this starting to make sense?

THE PROBLEM HERE IS THAT THERE IS ONLY ONE SEROTONIN MOLECULE, AND IT WILL "GO" TO THE RECEPTOR IT WISHES TO VISIT!

The technology does not exist at this time for the medical or pharmacological community to "make" serotonin "go" where medicine and pharmacy want it to "go." Nope! The body will decide just where that serotonin is needed (Hoyer, Hannon, & Martin, 2002).[9],[10]

Additionally, it is important to understand that there is no "correct level of serotonin." **There are no laboratory tests that can be used to diagnose depression or deficits in cognition, or migraines, or irritable bowel syndrome.**[11] There are also no correlations between the concentration of a specific medication in the bloodstream (or central nervous system) and therapeutic effect!

The only drug that blood levels are routinely used for clinical application would be lithium (discussed later in this book)- and the reason for those blood levels is the fact that the blood level that appears to be effective is very close to the blood level that is potentially fatal.[12]

The only thing "known" currently about serotonin levels in the body are that if a patient has elevate serotonin metabolites this may be indicative of the presence of a carcinoid tumor (Novartis Pharmaceuticals, 2013.)

Patients never state that they "feel their depression" in their synaptic space! All this once again solidifying the fact that all psychopharmacology is hypothetical!

So, the questions become "why are medications that are thought to work on neurotransmitters prescribed to patient with mental illnesses?" The answer is that for some patients who take these psychotropic

---

[9] The reference to Hoyer et al. about all the different 5HT receptors is a good one. This is one of the most complete descriptions of the diversity of serotonin receptor theory in research. The article is, candidly, much more that could be discussed coherently in a Primer, but note this quote from the article:

> However, the complexity of the system appears endless, since posttranslational modifications, such as alternate splicing and RNA editing, increase the number of proteins, oligomerisation and heteromerisation increase the number of complexes, and multiple G-protein suggest receptor trafficking, allowing phenotypic switching and crosstalk within and possibly between receptor families. **Whether all these possibilities are used in vivo under physiological or pathological conditions remains to be firmly established, but in essence, such variety will keep the 5-HT community busy for quite some time.** EMPHASIS ADDED. (Hoyer, Hannon, & Martin, 2002)

[10] Oh, indeed, this is why when a patient takes a medication- like an SSRI, an agonist- for mood disorders that patient may experience headaches, nausea, and vomiting. This means that there are other serotonin receptors that are being activated in addition to the ones thought to be involved in mood dysregulation.

[11] Coincidentally, the same statement applies to ALL neurotransmitters! That is why blood tests are never used as a diagnostic for mental health disorders.

[12] Some clinicians mistakenly state things like: "But there are blood draws for other mental health medications, like clozapine (Clozaril) or lamotrigine (Lamictal) or carbamazepine (Tegretol). This is true- but in these cases the blood draws are being done to assess other potential toxicities, like reduced white blood cell counts (clozapine), liver involvement (lamotrigine) or reduced red blood cells (carbamazepine).

medications, benefits, relief, and even sometimes remission are seen. When that happens, other patients with similar clinical presentations will then receive these medications.

While this may sound more than strange, consider this question:
"How does psychotherapy work?"

The chemistry of these neurotransmitters

Again, it is not within the scope of this book to teach the reader medicinal and organic chemistry. However, there are some aspects of chemistry that are needed to comprehend the significant aspects of neurotransmitter theory. And there are some really cool aspects of neurotransmitter biosynthesis that will help with understanding "why" certain drugs are used for specific conditions!

Begin with how the body "makes" serotonin:

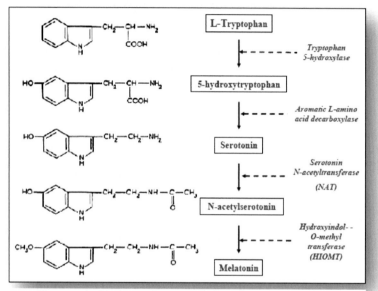

Chart used with the gracious permission of Peter A. Ensminger
(Ensminger, 2001)

Indeed, one of the "pathways" that the body uses to make serotonin begins with the amino acid tryptophan. One hears about tryptophan every Thanksgiving! This is the "Thanksgiving Turkey" chemical that is attributed to causing drowsiness.[13]

Note carefully that the body may ultimately use serotonin to make melatonin!

Oh, hang on, here! Is it not true that patients with depression often complain of sleep disturbances? Look in the DSM-IV TR or the DSM-5 and one will find under the diagnostic criteria for Major Depressive Disorder: "Insomnia or hypersomnia (*DSM-5*)". Perhaps the sleep disturbance is due to a dysregulation of the tryptophan-serotonin-melatonin biotransformation!

---

[13] This is a medical myth. There is no more tryptophan in turkey than there is in beef or chicken. The issue is not the tryptophan, but rather the quantity of food that is consumed at the Thanksgiving feast!

There is more, too. Indeed, when patients take medications that are thought to have an effect on serotonin levels (like selective serotonin reuptake inhibitors or serotonin/norepinephrine reuptake inhibitors) these patients sometimes complain of having trouble sleeping. Indeed, it is not uncommon to see a "sleeper" added to the patient's drug regimen. Perhaps by giving the patient medications that affect the serotonin-melatonin biotransformation pathway the prescriber is also causing a dysregulation in the "normal" biosynthesis.

Note carefully in the above flow chart that each neurotransmitter is affected by enzymes. Enzymes cause chemicals (and proteins) to change. There are indeed millions of enzymes, and many times the concept of enzymes becomes formidable and confusing. As the goal of this book is to make psychopharmacology "understandable" without "dumbing it down" here is a quick tip to help the reader understand enzymes:

ALL ENZYMES HAVE NAMES THAT END IN THE SUFFIX "-ASE."

All of them do. So there really is no need to memorize all the enzymes, just look for words in medicine and chemistry that end in "-ase." In the chart above, see that l-tryptophan is affected by the enzyme tryptophan 5-hydroxylase. Chemists would know that this means that an enzyme in the body has taken tryptophan and added a hydroxyl group (an oxygen atom attached to a hydrogen atom) at the "5" position of the tryptophan molecule. Look carefully at the chart above and you will see this.

But that is not the important construct in the theories of psychopharmacology and neurotransmitters. What is important is to know that the body used an enzyme (and the name of this enzyme ends with the suffix "-**ase**") to **change** tryptophan to 5-hydroxytryptophan. Even the names of the resulting chemicals (in this instance, "5-hydroxytryptophan") are not important- what is important is to know that the enzyme ("-**ase**") **changed** something in the body.

This is profoundly important. As an example, if a patient were to take a drug that prevented the enzyme from changing one chemical to a second chemical, then there would be "more" of that first chemical. That is why the drug class known as monoamine oxid**ase** inhibitors exists.

By preventing the enzyme monoamine oxid**ase** from changing any monoamine into another chemical, one would see an increase in that first chemical- the monoamine. And there are many monoamines- like serotonin, dopamine, epinephrine, and norepinephrine. That means that the antidepressants known as monoamine oxid**ase** inhibitors "work" by keeping serotonin, dopamine, epinephrine, and norepinephrine (all of these are thought to be neurotransmitters) from being "chewed up" so that there are "more" of these neurotransmitters.

This is also the reason that the monoamine oxid**ase** inhibitors (known in the industry as MAOIs) have problems with certain foods, like wine, cheese, etc. Wine and cheese (and the etc., by the way) all contain monoamines. The body likes keeping these monoamines "in balance" so the body uses monoamine oxid**ase** to "chew up" any monoamine that the body feels to be "in excess." Give a patient a MAOI? That patient has to be careful with dietary concerns.

So by preventing the change from serotonin to something else, one would find more serotonin available in the synaptic space! This concept, that by preventing enzymes from "chewing up" chemicals (including neurotransmitters), then there are more of those chemicals (including neurotransmitters) runs through the field of psychopharmacology and pharmacology. For instance, with Alzheimer's medications, one will find that drugs like donepezil (Aricept) are classified as acetylcholinester**ase** inhibitors! That means that donepezil (Aricept) prevents the enzyme acetylcholinester**ase** from "chewing up" or changing acetylcholine into something else, thereby resulting in increased acetylcholine levels.

AIDS patients often take prote**ase** inhibitors. These drugs prevent the enzyme prote**ase** from "chewing up" or changing protein!

Indeed, one could make an argument that any drug that increases the availability of a neurotransmitter is by definition an agonist (see previous chapter: "The concept of neurotransmitter activity".)

And now how the body makes dopamine, norepinephrine, and epinephrine- note that tis biochemical pathway is different from the one the body uses to make serotonin:

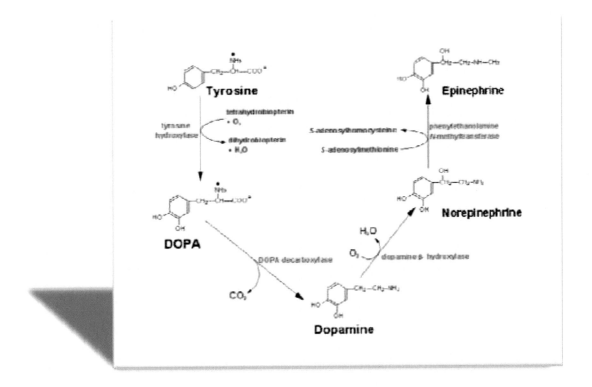

Graphic used with the kind permission of Michael W. King, Ph.D. (King, 2013).

Notice once again that **enzymes** are involved in the biotransformation of these chemicals.

There are some really interesting components in this biotransformation, too. Note that the body takes an amino acid (tyrosine) and uses an enzyme (tyrosine hydroxyl**ase**, see the "**-ase**" suffix, which means that the body is changing one chemical to another) to turn that tyrosine into dihydroxyphenylalanine.

Yes, dihydroxyphenylalanine is a really big word. And pharmacists, chemists, and medical folks do not like to use big words when acronyms will do. So in medicine, chemistry, and pharmacy, this chemical that the body produces from the amino acid tyrosine is known as DOPA (**D**ihydr**O**xy**P**henyl**A**lanine.)

DOPA was the drug that Dr. Oliver Sachs gave his patients found in the incredible book *Awakenings* (Sachs, 1999). This book was later made into a movie of the same title starring Robert De Niro and Robin Williams. Consider this- these patients were "frozen" (could not walk- or if they did, the patients had a "shuffle", often could not talk, had difficulty swallowing, had that odd "hand shaky thing"[14], could not

---

[14] The medical term for "hand shaky thing" is "extrapyramidal symptom", and is often represented by the abbreviation "EPS."

perform the most basic activities of daily living) due to their Parkinson's Disease.

Dr. Sachs felt that this condition was due to low levels of dopamine. Note in the chart above that the body uses enzymes to change DOPA into dopamine. Dr. Sachs gave those patients DOPA, which turned into dopamine (using enzymes), and the patients "awakened."

Too little dopamine[15] = Parkinson's.

But here is where it gets a little strange. Too MUCH dopamine[16] is thought to cause psychosis. More on that a little later in this book, but consider this- patients who take antipsychotic medications (which are thought to "work" as antagonists to dopamine) may have side effects that include that "hand shaky thing." Sometimes patients who take antipsychotics (again, dopamine antagonists) may sometimes have trouble swallowing, and have a robotic-like gait.

Again, **"TOO MUCH DOPAMINE"** activity= **PSYCHOSIS**. **"TOO LITTLE DOPAMINE"** activity= **PARKINSON'S DISEASE**.

There will be additional discussion about dopamine, dopamine agonists (increase dopamine activity), and dopamine antagonists (decrease dopamine activity) later in this book.

The reader will find that dopamine is also involved in other human experiences, notably pain, pleasure, and rage. But again, that is for a later discussion.

---

[15] This phrase: "Too little dopamine" must be construed to be a theoretical phrase only, as there is no "normal" dopamine level in the blood or the central nervous system.

[16] Ditto with the phrase "...too much dopamine." Just like in the previous footnote, this concept is hypothetical.

The concept of "normal" human activity and responses

O.K., now to focus on the "how and why" that these neurotransmitters exist in the human body. For this, it is necessary to look at some brain anatomy and some "normal" responses of the body. Brain anatomy is well beyond the scope of this book, and the reader is reminded that all this "science" is based on theoretical constructs. The goal of this short discussion on brain anatomy is to allow the reader to understand how the "fight or flight response" is based on theoretical underpinnings.

Begin with the AMYGDALA, a temporal lobe structure, which appears to be critical in assessing fear stimuli and danger response.

You've heard this as-

℞ Being the "Fight or Flight" response

Yes, some folks may have described this as a "Fight, Flight, Faint, Flop, or Freeze response...

But for purposes of this book, only the "Fight or Flight" response will be addressed.

The reason for this limitation? There are not any drugs that "mimic" the "Freeze" response! Well, given enough Thorazine....

The LOCUS CERULEUS is a structure on the brainstem, and is the primary norepinephrine depot on the brain. The LC has pathways into areas that seem to implement the fear responses, like the VAGUS NERVE; as well as the LATERAL and PARAVENTRICULAR HYPOTHALAMUS.

Ah, the vagus nerve! This cranial nerve innervates the heart, the lungs, and the intestines- those organs over which a person has no control. On 06/15/2004 the FDA's Neurological Advisory Panel recommended APPROVAL of the vagus nerve stimulator as a treatment for chronic depression![17]

But at the end of 2004, the FDA denied this recommendation (this treatment has since been approved by the FDA.) There may have been some possible reasons for the denial in 2004[18] notably that the FDA may have had too much on its plate:

- There was no resident Director of the FDA
- Suicide problems with SSRIs were a significant issue (10/04)

---

[17] The vagal nerve stimulator has been approved by the FDA to treat epilepsy since 1997. Note that this is used for MOOD as well as for seizures. More on this concept- mood disorders and seizures- as this book continues.

[18] This is now FDA approved for patients 18 years of age or older with treatment resistant depression.

- There were testing integrity concerns with several drug applications
- There was a flu vaccine shortage
- Politics

Now, back to brain stuff. The ENTORHINAL CORTEX is the main interface between the hippocampus and neocortex. The ENTORHINAL CORTEX-HIPPOCAMPAL system plays an important role in autobiographical/declarative/episodic memories, and in particular, spatial memories including memory formation, memory consolidation, and memory optimization in sleep (Wikipedia, 2013).

The entorhinal cortex is the most primitive part of your brain, and is the seat of the sense of smell.[19] Consider this- when you were a caveperson, out hunting and gathering, you might not see a saber-toothed tiger, as that creature was camouflaged; you might not hear that creature, as that creature is stealthy. But you would certainly SMELL that tiger and then take actions to survive.

The HIPPOCAMPUS is pivotal in consolidating traumatic memory and with the entorhinal cortex is relative for fear conditioning, which is thought to be involved in chronic anxiety. The HYPOTHALAMUS (the "master gland") integrates neuroendocrine and autonomic threat responses. This, dear reader, leads to the fact that one cannot- repeat CANNOT- separate hormones from neurotransmitters in any logical discussion. The focus of this book, however, is not endocrinology, but rather psychopharmacology. There will be additional references to hormones in this book, however.[20]

O.K., so that concept of how the brain gets involved is a little clearer. Look again, though, at that chart on page 25 that describes how the body changes tyrosine into DOPA and then into dopamine, then into norepinephrine, and finally into epinephrine. Recall that this is the "fight or flight" response.

Any drug that affects dopamine could "change" the clinical presentation of patients. Consider this theory:

Dopamine is the "fight" of the fight or flight response; norepinephrine is the "flight."

So any drug that increases the activity of dopamine (agonism) could increase the "fight." It is not uncommon to see patients who use cocaine, crystal methamphetamine, Ecstasy (or the derivative known on the street as "Molly" or "Mandy") and yes, even prescription medications like Adderall and Ritalin to have increased levels of hostility- although in the medical and psychological fields this would be called "increased psychomotor effect." Giving the patient an antipsychotic medication like

---

[19] This is why aromatherapy may be of benefit- and possibly detriment- to patients (Smith, 2014.)

[20] Reflect that when one is being chased by a tiger, the brain also releases cortisol- also known as "stress hormone."

Abilify, Risperdal, or Thorazine (dopamine antagonists) would reduce that "fight."

But wait, there's more to this neurotransmitter dopamine! Dopamine is also involved in the "pleasure", "pain", and "rage" responses. Indeed, people need dopamine to have orgasms (pleasure); drugs like the opioids (codeine, heroin, morphine, etc.) also affect the dopamine system (pain, possibly some of the pleasure experience...more on this later in this book); and the "ragefulness" is also thought to be mediated by dopamine activity. One cannot rape and pillage without dopamine! This is why both sides of the World War II conflict were given doses of amphetamine- to make them channel the rage, to make the combatants better killing machines (Center for Substance Abuse Research- University of Maryland, 2013) . The combatants were able to focus on their targets, and become more efficient.

Wait a minute, here! Amphetamines used in wartime helped people focus? Then...why not give amphetamines to people who difficulty in focusing? Like people with Attention Deficit/Hyperactivity Disorder?

And that is why to this day the drugs amphetamine, dextroamphetamine, methylphenidate, etc., are used today to treat ADHD! That is also the reason that some patients who use dopamine agonists- everything from cocaine to Adderall to medications used for treatment of Parkinson's Disease- may have psychological presentations that could include rage.

Oh, continue with that chart on page 25, and note that the dopamine is changed into norepinephrine. On the previous page, it was noted that norepinephrine is the "flight" of the fight or flight response. Indeed, if one is in a stressful situation, like, for instance, being placed in the path of a saber-toothed tiger, one would try to run away!

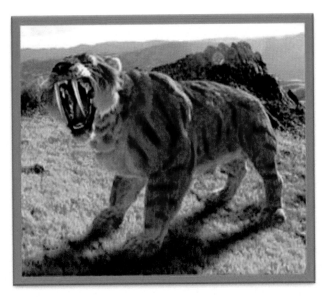

The person who encountered this sabre toothed tiger would experience a fast heart rate and very shallow breathing, all due to the increased levels of norepinephrine the brain is causing to happen in response to this dangerous meeting with this predator. Running away requires an increase in the heart rate and more oxygen to the muscles. This is the β-adrenergic system kicking in. So, if one wanted to REDUCE the β-adrenergic activity, one would give the patient a β-blocker (a β-adrenergic antagonist.)

This is why these medications- the "β-blockers" are used to treat heart dysrhythmias and high blood pressure (these medications cause the blood vessels to relax, due to decreased sympathetic tone.)

Now, consider what a person often experiences as a result of anxiety:

Feeling of apprehension, dread	Difficulty in concentrating
Hypervigilance (being on the lookout for danger)	Catastrophizing ("I'm going to be eaten!")
Restlessness	Irritability
Feeling tense, or "jumpy	"Zoning out"
A pounding of the heart	Muscle tension

Administration of a β-blocker would offset these components of anxiety! A more detailed discussion of the use of the β-blockers to treat anxiety will happen later in this book.

Now you, gentle reader, know just exactly why β-blockers are sometime used for treatment of anxiety. By the way, performance artists sometimes use the β-blocker propranolol before giving a presentation, known as "performance anxiety"- as these medications would offset "stage fright "or "the butterflies" (truly a cardiac dysrhythmia).

Hey, something else to consider! When that person is being chased by a saber toothed tiger, is that patient depressed? Absolutely not!

Gee...if there were to be a drug that makes a person feel like he or she is being chased by a saber toothed tiger, then that drug could be used to treat depression!

And here is why the tricyclic medications like Elavil, Tofranil, and even the tetracyclic medication Remeron, are used to treat depression! Indeed, these medications are thought to cause an increase in norepinephrine (increasing the "tiger response"- an agonistic activity!) Reflect, too, that the patients who use tricyclic and/or tetracyclic antidepressants may be at risk for cardiac dysrhythmias!

This is another of the pillars of psychopharmacology, and why psychopharmacology should not be that "hard"- look at what the body does "normally" as a response and then either increase or decrease that response! Focus on the body's "normal response" and give an agonist (to increase that response) or an antagonist (to decrease that response.)

That, truly, is the _SECRET OF PSYCHOPHARMACOLOGY_- and pharmacology- in general.

Now to address the science of pharmacology- literally: the study of drugs in the human body

Drugs "work" by several different "mechanisms."

It is thought that the active compounds in medicines affect how the body works by interacting with the substances in and around cells.

And, sometimes, the "inactive compounds" may have an effect!

These "mechanisms"...

Affect the chemical processes which keep the body healthy and working properly.

Three ways that these interactions are important:

1. Medicines may affect the whole body or organ system in a general way
2. Medicines may be specific and affect only a particular part of the body
3. Medicines may replace or repair defective genes to treat disease (called gene therapy)

Understand that there are no "pediatric drugs" or "geriatric drugs." In the United States, there are drugs which are approved for use for certain CLINICAL INDICATIONS. That means that if a drug is approved for, say, "depression" then it may be used for treating that clinical condition...

...even if the drug has not been tested in specific populations, like:

- o Children
- o Pregnant clients
- o Nursing mothers
- o Elderly folks
- o Immunocompromised individuals
- o Etc.

Drugs are tested on "young, healthy" people, as a rule. This is a problem as drugs are not always meant to be used only on "young, healthy people."

"No Magic Pill"[21] for treating symptoms of Alzheimer's, study finds" (Mesure, 2005).

The study, published in *The Journal of the American Medical Association*, found that antidepressants such as Prozac and mood stabilizers such as Tegretol offer little or no relief for the behavioral symptoms of Alzheimer's.

> *"These drugs were designed for younger patients and not for older Alzheimer's patients,' says William Thies of the Chicago-based Alzheimer's Association.*

---

[21] Remember the discussion of the "Magic Bullet" earlier in this book, and the history of when penicillin was developed? See page 11.

31

But doctors are under enormous pressure to prescribe drugs to treat such behaviors. 'Caregivers want a magic pill,' says Kaycee Sink, lead author of the paper. "What our study showed is that there is no magic pill.'" (Mesure, 2005)

Indeed, a drug may carry-

A warning stating that the use of the drug during pregnancy is "contraindicated."

A "Black Box Warning" informing the prescriber that the drug may have specific dangers, <u>but that does not mean that the drug cannot be used in pediatric, adolescent, or geriatric populations</u>, even though there are significant homeostatic variables within these different age, gender and ethnic groups. (The topic of "homeostasis" will be mentioned again in this book, several times.)

The use of drugs in the elderly, for example:

People aged 65 and over are seriously underrepresented in clinical drug trials, even though as a class this group takes the most medications! As example, women over the age of 65, who account for almost half of all cases of breast cancer, constituted only 9% of clinical trial participants (Kemeny, 2003)!

Why is this?

If the FDA were to tell drug companies that a drug would not be approved until the drug company provided data on a specific group (say, people between the age of 75 and 85) the pharmaceutical companies would have to spend more money in the research stage.

And this is a problem because....

Researchers may consider children, old folks, disabled folks, etc., to be to "frail" or will exclude people who have comorbid disease states from the clinical trials, but then the researchers do not learn what makes these classes of patients' physiologies unique.

Drugs may be used to treat "other" conditions...
- That is why we use blood pressure medications to treat anxiety
- Or antinauseants to treat psychosis
- Or .....

Remember, once a drug is "approved" it is allowed to be prescribed for any condition the prescriber feels appropriate.

What about those "other" uses of drugs? Well, "Off Label" uses are "allowed." Aspirin for preventing heart attacks, for instance, was only recently "approved." Prozac had been shown to help Obsessive Compulsive Disorder (OCD) and panic disorder, but only recently was labeling changed to show this as "approved."

But "fen-phen" was ALSO an "off-label" use, which had fatal results. And now some prescribers are using "phen-pro" for weight reduction therapy, which is phentermine and fluoxetine (Prozac), and, you guessed it, this is not an FDA approved combination.

The FDA and Congress are the drivers behind this. Yes, indeed, a little more history about how psychological, medical, and pharmacological industries have arrived at "off-label" or unapproved uses of prescription medications.

The original 1938 Federal Food, Drug and Cosmetic Act required that all drugs be proven "safe" before they could be marketed for human use. In 1962, Congress required that the FDA mandate that these drugs also be "effective."

So now, the FDA says a drug must be "safe and effective." Note: not "better" than any other treatment (not even better than placebo!) just "safe and effective."

And this meant that the labeling of the drugs can only state uses that have been FDA approved for selected populations and for specific doses. Then, in 1997, the Congress enacted the FDA Modernization Act, which contained a provision that would allow drug manufacturers to "disseminate information about unapproved uses of drugs…"

This "dissemination of information" would include peer-reviewed journal articles of "off-label" uses, if the pharmaceutical manufacturer committed itself to file, within a specified time frame, a supplemental application based on appropriate research to establish safety and effectiveness.

U.S. District Judge Royce C. Lamberth ruled in 1999, however, that this "requirement" to file a supplemental application was UNCONSTITUTIONAL because it violated the First Amendment by restricting the right to commercial free speech. (FindLaw for Legal Professionals, 2008)

Here's how the ruling was interpreted…the pharmaceutical companies construed this ruling rather narrowly, and now may distribute "a medical journal" to a physician as long as that medical journal is "not false or misleading" and as long as the pharmaceutical company discloses the company's interest in the drug.

Scary, huh?

The United States Senate Passed S.B. 650 on July 24, 2003- the Pediatric Research Equity Act of 2003, (Govtrack.us, 2003) giving FDA the authority to perform pediatric testing on certain products. Note well, however, that this bill would require drug manufacturers "to assess the safety and effectiveness of the drug or biological product for the claimed indications in all relevant PEDIATRIC subpopulations."

S.B. 650 specifically prohibited that safety and effectiveness expansion to other patient populations! Like adolescents, for instance? Like the aged population, perhaps?

S.B. 650 was referred to the United States House of Representatives on July 23, 2003 and was signed by President George W. Bush in December 2003 as Public Law 108-155.

"Medications often given to children have been deemed safe only for use by adults" (USA Today, 2003)."

WASHINGTON- The government announced plans to begin clinical trials on 12 drugs commonly prescribed for children even though their safety and effectiveness has been tested only in adults.

Here are the 12 drugs that will be tested in clinical trials for use by children and what they treat:

- *Azithromycin: An antibiotic used to treat many different types of bacterial infection.*
- *Baclofen: A muscle relaxant used to relieve the spasms and tightness caused by such problems as multiple sclerosis or certain injuries to the spine.*
- *Bumetanide: Used to reduce the swelling and fluid retention caused by various medical problems, including heart or liver disease. It also is used to treat high blood pressure.*
- *Dobutamine: A heart stimulating drug.*
- *Dopamine: Used to treat Parkinson's and schizophrenia.*
- *Furosemide: Used to treat swelling and water retention.*
- *Heparin: Used to decrease the clotting ability of the blood and help prevent harmful clots from forming in the blood vessels*
- *Lithium: Treatment for bipolar disorder.*
- *Lorazepam: Treatment for anxiety.*
- *Rifampin: Used in combination with other medications to treat tuberculosis, and to treat carriers of meningitis-causing bacteria.*
- *Sodium Nitroprusside: A treatment for high blood pressure.*
- *Spironolactone: A treatment for high blood pressure.*

Remember, too, that a single drug may have different uses.

This book will address the major clinical indication of the drugs; lesser-used indications may also be discussed, just as the psychotherapies may be used for different conditions. For example, Progressive Relaxation therapy can benefit not only those patients who have anxiety, but also those with depression, insomnia, headaches, Post-Traumatic Stress Disorder (PTSD), or a "mixture" of diagnostic conditions.

So, for this book-

The reader will see drugs that are used in children, adolescents, adults, and the elderly, the infirm.

And the format will be-

- ℞ To discuss the drugs by class
- ℞ To discuss the chemical structures, and why structures these are important in finding out how the drugs work in the body
- ℞ To discuss the pharmacology of the drugs
- ℞ To see some of the ethical problems surrounding the employment of these

Note that ALL drugs in ALL groups will not be discussed. After all, this book is indeed intended to be a "primer." Also note that in this book discussion will be about the <u>commonly</u> encountered mental health conditions, and <u>common</u> psychological diagnoses that might result in the prescribing of psychoactive drugs.

The goal will be to understand which drugs ***MAY BE CONSIDERED*** as therapeutic agents for these clinical conditions.

The disclaimer...[22]

Nothing in this presentation, this book, or the resources listed, as well as the opinions of Thomas A. Smith should be in any way considered to be suggestive of implementation or discontinuation of any current, proposed, or future therapy as being appropriate for consumers of this book, family members of persons reading this book, patients of persons who read this book, strangers that anyone who might read this book might meet, people that readers of this book know, pets of people reading this book, the pets of neighbors of persons who read this book, or anyone at all.

Any questions regarding health should always be directed to a competent health practitioner.

Readers of this book are aware of the nature of the contents of this presentation and program and do not now, nor will you in the future hold Thomas A. Smith, Smith Rehabilitation Consultants, Inc., employees/staff/consultants, or others involved with the printing, editing, distribution, administration, presentation, and implementation of this book responsible at law or in equity for any emotional, mental, psychological, physical, developmental, or other stresses or harm that readers of this book, any patients of persons who read this book, family members of persons who read this book, any person with whom readers of this book might discuss this book, the practice of anyone reading this book, etc., may experience during or after reading this book.

There will be no specific discussion of "dosages" in this book. This may sound odd to readers of this primer, but there is a specific reason for not including dosages, although some medications will have doses listed when the information is pertinent to the understanding of the reader.

The "correct" dose of mental health medication is based upon the needs of the individuals taking those drugs, the risk *vs.* benefit of the medications, the patient's therapeutic response, co-morbid disease states, co-administered medications, and the prescriber's clinical decisions.

Last, when the reader sees a trade or patented or trademarked or registered drug name for convenience the little attendant symbols appertaining to those medications are not included[23]...all the drugs in this book are either Copyrighted, Patented, and/or Trademarked by their respective owner (s).

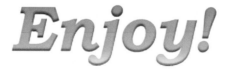

---

[22] Stuff our lawyer makes us put in this book!
[23] Such things as the symbols: ®, ™, ©, etc.

Antianxiety treatments-the anxiolytics...

Yes, there are many different types of treatments that have been used to treat anxiety states. "Anxiolytic" means "dissolves anxiety."

Let's review... chemical treatments for anxiety (and insomnia):

- ℞ Barbiturates
- ℞ Benzodiazepines
- ℞ Non-benzodiazepines

These can be used for "nerves" or to induce sleep...

Begin with the herbals, treatments that date back to antiquity. It was not uncommon for someone who was "stressed" to be told to "take a tea." Some of these teas would include chamomile and kava kava, but even warm milk has been used to relieve anxiety.

The goal of anxiolytics, or "nerve pills," is also to reduce anxiety.

The barbiturates-

These drugs are rarely, if ever, used anymore, but that does not mean that clinicians will never encounter them in clinical practice with children, adolescents, or the elderly populations.

Some of these drugs are ancient-Developed by Adolph Bayer in the 1860's (yes, he of "Bayer Aspirin" fame.) The barbiturates were first marketed in 1903, and there were over 50 developed.

What were the barbiturates originally used for?

- Anxiety;
- Grief;
- Depression (more on this concept later- the use of anti-anxiety medications to treat depression as well as the use of anti-depressant medications to treat anxiety); and,
- Seizures

What are they used for now?

- To control seizures;
- As an IV anesthetic;
- To produce sedation in emergencies or in therapy;
- To reduce brain activity, blood flow and release of glutamate after severe head injury (as example, "drug-induced coma states");
- In capital executions;
- In assisted suicides; and,
- For inducing sleep

There are differences (and similarities) between the barbiturates[24]-

---

[24] Note well- not all of these barbiturate medications are still being marketed in the United States, and not all the barbiturates are listed below.

Butabarbital (Butisol)
Mephobarbital (Mebaral)
Luminal (Phenobarbital)
Amobarbital (Amytal)
Secobarbital (Secanol)

Aprobarbital (Alurate)
Methohexital (Brevital)
Sodium thiopental (Sodium
Pentothal)

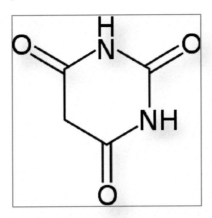

The chemical structure above is the "chemical chassis" that is shared by ALL barbiturates.
This is known as "barbituric acid."
Minor changes to this "chassis" yields the different medications known as the "barbiturates."

How do the barbiturates work?

First, the "general depressant" effects are indistinguishable from alcohol, and the depressant effects are due to increasing the inhibitory effects of GABA (gamma amino butyric acid) – GABA is an inhibitory neurotransmitter. Throughout this book, GABA will be called "**THE BRAKES OF THE BRAIN.**"

Higher doses of barbiturates may affect other neurotransmitters, too.

GABA is the main inhibitory neurotransmitter in the Central Nervous System (CNS), and GABA is involved in nerve transmission in nearly 33% of brain impulses. This is an important number, because if GABA affected 100% of the brain impulses, any person who was to take barbiturates would die.

The GABA system has strong regulatory and/or inhibitory effects on the 5-HT (serotonin) and NE (norepinephrine) systems. This is why a patient who takes a barbiturate might experience depression as a side effect.

There are different GABA receptors, which may produce different pharmacological (and clinical) effects/ GABA binds to three principal receptors, each of which is involved in different physiologic functions.

$GABA_A$ receptors- mediate fast inhibitory synaptic transmissions. $GABA_A$ receptors are thought to regulate neuronal excitability (such as seizure threshold) and rapid changes in mood. $GABA_A$ receptors are the "targets" of benzodiazepines, barbiturates, and ethanol.

GABA$_B$ receptors- mediate slow inhibitory potentials (the electricity in the cells); GABA$_B$ receptors appear to be important in memory, mood, and pain.

GABA$_C$ receptors- well, researchers are not so sure about these

Their physiologic (maybe psychological?) role has not yet been fully described. And there may be more GABA receptors that have not been found yet...

Here is how medications may be used to affect GABA:

GABAergic activity may be enhanced by either:

- ❖ <u>Stimulating</u> GABA$_A$ receptors (GABA$_A$-receptor agonists or modulating compounds)
- ❖ <u>Inhibition</u> of GABA metabolism
- ❖ <u>Direct inhibition</u> of GABA <u>reuptake</u> from the synapse by blocking the action of GATs (selective GABA-reuptake inhibitors)

And now a discussion about GABA transporter protein, also known as "GATs": GATs are membrane-transporter proteins that remove GABA from the synaptic cleft. Four distinct GATs have been identified:

- ❖ GAT-1, GAT-2, GAT-3, and BGT-1

These GATs are found on neurons, both pre- and postsynaptically, and on glial cells, and differ in CNS distribution and localization. As example, GAT-1 is the primary GABA transporter in the brain, and the density of GAT-1 is highest in the frontal and parietal cortex of the brain.

GABA "turns on" blockade-

It is believed that barbiturates effectively "turn on" this blockade, by making GABA bind to the GABA receptor. In essence, GABA works by blocking the cell from "doing what it would normally do." This means, that if a medication will "increase" GABA, then the body would "shut down" excitation of the neural pathways.

This is what barbiturates are thought to "do."

As one might expect, there can be problems with the use of barbiturates. Withdrawal begins with growing anxiety, agitation, "the shakes", GI upset and bodily arousal.[25]

Severe withdrawal includes delirium, seizures, uncontrolled heart rhythm and possible death, even with medical supervision. Dose-dependent withdrawal is very similar to alcohol withdrawal and is characterized by hyperexcitability of body and brain.[26]

---

[25] Note how this sounds an awful lot like DT's: *Delirium Tremens*, alcohol withdrawal.

[26] Consider that the use of barbiturates "shut down" activity- like "putting the brakes on the brain." That would mean that REMOVING the barbiturates would allow the brain to have unfettered activity, similar to driving down a mountain after the "brakes" of the car have burned out.

The Benzodiazepines-

These are also known as "minor tranquilizers"- and the hypnotic benzodiazepines are known as "sleepers."

So just how do benzodiazepines (BZDs) work? Remember the GABA inhibition of the barbiturates?

The "Benzodiazepine Receptor Model" is based on the premise that there is a link between the GABA type A (GABA$_A$) receptor and a chloride ion channel. When this happens, the chloride ion channel opens, allowing negatively charged chloride ions to influx into the cell membrane, causing hyperpolarization, which results in a decrease in nerve excitability.

Right about now, after that previous paragraph, the reader is possibly thinking: "What?"

What this means is that the "brakes of the brain" have been turned on (the GABA) and the cell has been "short-circuited."

Benzodiazepines have some benefits over barbiturates; notably, BZDs have an antagonist available, where there is no antagonist available for the barbiturates. This BZD antagonist is known as flumazenil (Romazicon[27]) and is thought to have a mechanism of action that allows binding with the receptor without opening the ion channel. When this happens, there is a further blocking to the receptor by GABA. Literally this is "blocking the blocking" that GABA could cause.

Benzodiazepines are used for anxiety states, such as (there are others, too!):

Panic Attack	Specific Phobia	Separation Anxiety	Agoraphobia
Panic Disorder Without Agoraphobia	Anxiety Disorder Due to Another Medical Condition		Panic Attack With Agoraphobia
Obsessive-Compulsive Disorder	Post-Traumatic Stress Disorder		Agoraphobia Without History of Panic Disorder
Acute Stress Disorder	Generalized Anxiety Disorder		Social Phobia
Substance-Induced Anxiety Disorder		Other Specified Anxiety Disorder	

---

[27] Flumazenil, when used to treat benzodiazepine overdose may precipitate life-threatening seizures. Many poison control centers and emergency rooms no longer even consider using flumazenil for suspected cases of BZD overdose, especially if the patient has a history of benzodiazepine-tolerance. If the patient has been using BZDs for a long time, then care should be employed before considering using flumazenil, as often all that is necessary is to wait out the overdose by using supportive measures, such as monitoring and treating vital signs.

These benzodiazepine medications are also used to induce sleep. Because there are significant chemical similarities between the benzodiazepines[28], the "sleepers" will be presented right along with the "minor tranquilizers" in this book, as well as the benzodiazepine medications usually used as anticonvulsants.

The difference between sleepers and "minor tranquilizer" benzodiazepines?

How long the individual drug produces a clinical effect in the body!

See the chart on page 44!

Remember, however, that benzodiazepine may be used for both clinical conditions- anxiety and sleep. These medications are also used to treat seizures, as BZDs "put the brakes on the brain."

What BZDs do:

℞ Alleviate the anxiety state

℞ Resolve "tension"

℞ Cause sedation

What a clinician might expect from a patient's clinical presentation after the patient uses a benzodiazepine:

℞ A "calmer" client

---

[28]Here are just a few examples of the chemical structures of benzodiazepines. Note how these have the same "chassis": - the similarity of the structure. This is why all these medications belong to the drug or chemical "class" known as benzodiazepines. This "similarity of chemical structure" is presented throughout this book. This is one of the "ways" in which chemicals are "classified' as members of a specific chemical "family."

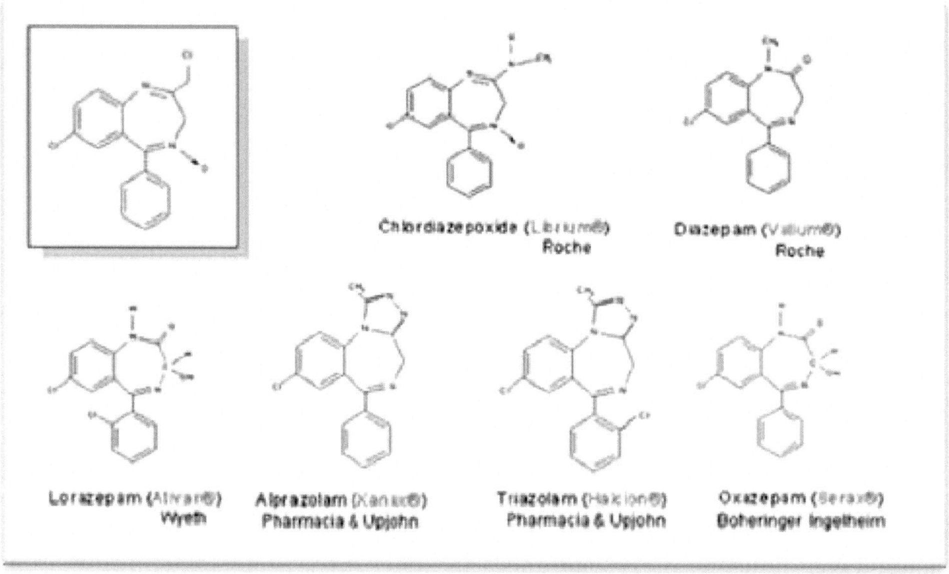

Chlordiazepoxide (Librium®)
Roche

Diazepam (Valium®)
Roche

Lorazepam (Ativan®)
Wyeth

Alprazolam (Xanax®)
Pharmacia & Upjohn

Triazolam (Halcion®)
Pharmacia & Upjohn

Oxazepam (Serax®)
Boheringer Ingelheim

Problems that might be encountered with the use of the benzodiazepine medications (regardless of whether the BZD is used for treatment of anxiety, sleep, or to treat seizures):

- Addiction liability
- Dizziness, drowsiness, blurred vision
- Overdose
  - Either intentional or otherwise

Here are a few of the more commonly encountered benzodiazepine medications:

Benzodiazepines (some Brand names in the United States)[29] BZDs usually used to treat insomnia are *italicized*, but remember these all have the same "mechanism of action." The "sleepers" will be discussed later in this book.	Half-life, in hours, of the drug and of the active metabolite of the drug.[30]	The approximate oral milligram dosage equivalent, one benzodiazepine to another on this list. Note that these dosages might be considered on the "high side" of the therapeutic range normally prescribed.
Alprazolam (Xanax)	6-12	0.5
Chlordiazepoxide (Librium)	5-40 (36-200)	25
Clonazepam (Klonopin)[31]	18-50	0.5
Clorazepate (Tranxene)	(36-200)[32]	15
Diazepam (Valium)	20-100 (36-200)	10
***Estazolam*[33]**	10-24	1-2
Flunitrazepam (Rohypnol)[34]	18-26 (36-200)	1
***Flurazepam* (Dalmane)**	(40-250)[23]	15-30
Lorazepam (Ativan)	10-20	1
Oxazepam	4-15	20
***Quazepam* (Doral)**	25-100	20
***Temazepam* (Restoril)**	8-22	20
***Triazolam* (Halcion)**	2	0.5

Because these medications are so similar in chemical structure this book will focus only on one:

Alprazolam (Xanax).

This is a triazolobenzodiazepine[35], or for the technical folks this is a triazolo analog of the 1,4 benzodiazepine class.

---

[29] Note well that there are quite a few other benzodiazepam drugs available throughout the world. This reference is only for those benzodiazepine medications currently available in the United States at the time of the publishing of this book in early 2014.

[30] The half-life of a drug, for this book, is defined as the time taken for blood concentration to fall to half its peak value after a single dose. Again, for this book, the half-lives of active metabolites are shown in parenthetical brackets. The half-life times may vary considerably between individuals, due to such things a liver health, body mass, genetics, co-morbid physical conditions, interactions with other drugs or food, etc.

[31] Clonazepam is technically used as an antiseizure medication, but in mental health this medication is often seen being employed to treat chronic anxieties.

[32] Clorazepate and flurazepam are known in pharmacy as a "pro-drugs." These medications have no effect on its own, but rather must be metabolized into an active metabolite before a therapeutic effect may be seen.

[33] Estazolam and oxazepam are only available in the United States as generic products. The brand names- ProSom for estazolam and Serax for oxazepam- have been removed from the market.

[34] See next section. This drug is not officially available in the United States, and it is considered an illegal drug in the US.

Alprazolam is usually prescribed to treat anxiety, and is indicated for short-term treatment. This medication is also used to treat anxiety associated with depression, as well as to treat panic. Alprazolam has an "unlabeled" use to treat agoraphobia, and is used to premenstrual syndrome (PMS) as well as a treatment for depression.[36]

Drug comparisons:

Alprazolam is known as a benzodiazepine with high potency, rapid distribution, and is short-acting. Due to the short-acting nature of this drug it is not usually a good choice for anxiety disorders, due to:

- Rebound effect
- Difficulty in covering a 24-hour period without very frequent dosing

Finishing alprazolam (Xanax), after a rapid decrease in dosage or abrupt discontinuation of this drug, there may be withdrawal seizures. Anger, hostility and episodes of mania and hypomania have been reported with this drug, and there have been reports of coma in patients taking both Xanax and Kava Kava.

---

[35] This long chemical name is mentioned only so that the reader may appreciate that there are many similar medications. As example, the antipsychotic medication olanzapine (Zyprexa) is classified as a thieno**benzodiazepine**.

[36] This may surprise the reader, that a drug that is usually used to treat anxiety might also be used to treat depression. Understand that in the Diagnostic and Statistical Manual of Mental Disorders, 5th Edition, (DSM-5, 2013) about 55% of the diagnostic criteria for anxiety are shared with depression.

Somnotics (also known as "hypnotics") – these are the "sleepers"

Should not patients who have insomnia receive treatment? This is a philosophical question- and the question should require some more information. As example:

- Are there underlying pathologies, either physical or psychological?
    - Is the insomnia a symptom of depression?
    - Is the insomnia a symptom of anxiety?
- Could the patient be having sleep problems as a result of PTSD?
- Is there a tumor that is affecting the brain?
- Is the patient in chronic pain?
- Could there be substance abuse?
    - Do not forget caffeine here!
- Is this possibly a "situational" insomnia?
    - Noisy neighbors
    - Road construction
- Is there use and abuse of over-the-counter medications?

Here is a protocol regarding the use of somnotics, from the author of this book:

The best treatment is the least treatment, if at all

- ℞ Warm milk (human breast milk contains lots of tryptophan)
- ℞ Jergen's Baby Lavender Bath (use in the bath, not as a lotion)
- ℞ Have no exercise for at least 4 hours before bedtime
- ℞ Consider changing environmental aspects of the bedroom (in psychotherapy this is called "sleep hygiene")

Room temperature	Get a better pillow
Get a better mattress	Turning off "blue lights"
Turning off the television, radio, cellphone, computer	

- ℞ Doing something really boring instead of just lying in bed
    - Balance your checkbook
- ℞ Pray
    - Reading the 10th Chapter of Genesis in the *Bible* is good- that is the "begat chapter"
    - Judges and Deuteronomy are also good chapters in the *Bible* to put one to sleep

DO NOT READ THE "REVELATIONS" CHAPTER IN THE *BIBLE* BEFORE GOING TO BED!

- Sometimes it is better to not count sheep, but talk to the Shepherd (if one is a person of certain faiths)
- ℞ Meditate
- ℞ Possibly using some α-brain wave stimulation

This protocol is not bad for anxiety, ADHD, and migraine headaches, either!

Then, if there has been no improvement in insomnia, *maybe* somnotics FOR SHORT-TERM USE!

Look at a few (not all) of the benzodiazepines that are used as sleepers, followed by the "non-benzodiazepine" prescription medications

These benzodiazepine sleepers again are drugs of the same "class" as Xanax, Librium, Ativan, etc., previously discussed in this book. Just like in that section of this book, not all the sleepers will be discussed, as they all have the same mechanism of action and all share the basic chemical structure of the BZDs.

Temazepam (Restoril)
Classification: Sedative/hypnotic, benzodiazepine (BZD)
Used as: Somnotic
Temazepam has a rapid to intermediate onset of action, with a wide distribution throughout the system, and a relatively short half-life. All of these have made this medication one where the client can get to sleep quickly, but without much of a "hangover" effect. If a patient has some problems with liver disease, temazepam is relatively safe (United States National Library of Medicine: National Institute of Diabetes and Digestive and Kidney Diseases, 2013). Temazepam is very similar to oxazepam (Serax) – a BZD used for anxiety- in this aspect.

Triazolam (Halcion)
Classification: Sedative/hypnotic, benzodiazepine (BZD)
Used as: Somnotic
Triazolam has high potency, rapid distribution, and is short-acting. This medication is used in "sedation dentistry",
There are some claims that this drug causes higher dependence than other BZDs (this drug has been outlawed in Great Britain and Brazil as a result of those claims) (Adam & Oswald, 1993). The risk is controversial (Manfredi & Kales, 1987).
Clients have been reported to wake up earlier in the morning with triazolam than with other intermediate- or long-acting somnotics. This is why triazolam is used in "sedation dentistry."
Due to the short-acting nature of this drug it is obviously not a good choice for anxiety disorders, due to:
℞ Rebound effect
℞ Difficulty in covering a 24-hour period without very frequent dosing

These next three drugs (in this book) are not "technically" benzodiazepines...

...but are believed to work in that GABA-chloride ion channel complex just like the benzodiazepines (Librium, Valium, Xanax) do, but their chemical structure is markedly different- these drugs do not have that shared "chassis" described earlier.

Zolpidem (Ambien, Intermezzo, Zolipmist)
Classification: Somnotic-hypnotic, imidazopyridine
Used as: Somnotic
Zolpidem is indicated for short-term treatment like all sleepers (7-10 days) but it is not uncommon to see patients using this medication on a more routine, even sometimes every night dosing schedule. It is recommended that the client should be re-evaluated if this drug is needed for longer periods of time, obviously to rule out other causes of the insomnia.

The short half-life of zolpidem may be advantageous, in that a patient may fall asleep quickly; however, patients using zolpidem have been known to wake up halfway through the night.

It is suggested that the mode of action is a subunit modulation of the GABA receptor chloride channel macromolecular complex

Dosage concerns with zolpidem would include that the elderly or debilitated client may be especially sensitive to the effects of this drug. As a matter of fact, patients with hepatic insufficiency may not be able to clear this drug as rapidly as healthy patients; indeed, in January 2013 the FDA issued new dosage guidelines, specifically that women should be dosed at half the dose usually used in men, due to metabolic differences.

Zolpidem is chemically unrelated to the BZDs; however, it is included in the discussion of this class of drugs as it has a high affinity for type 1 benzodiazepine receptors, as do zaleplon (Sonata) and eszopiclone (Lunesta).

Zaleplon (Sonata)
Classification: Somnotic.

Used as: Somnotic-hypnotic; Indicated for the treatment of short-term insomnia.

Zaleplon is rapidly and almost completely absorbed following oral administration (food may slow this down.) Peak plasma levels are seen within an hour, and zaleplon has a short half-life of about an hour. Like zolpidem, zaleplon is also is thought to interact with the GABA receptor chloride channel macromolecular complex.

Dosing concerns with zaleplon (Sonata) may sound similar to what was seen with zolpidem, in that the elderly or debilitated client may be especially sensitive to the effects of this drug. Of note is that with zaleplon (Sonata) Japanese clients seem to have higher concentrations of this drug (37% higher)

(Donaldson, Gizzarelli, & Chanpong, 2007), which may be due to body weight or enzymatic activity.

Eszopiclone (Lunesta)

While not a benzodiazepine, the action of this drug is: "…believed to result from its interaction with GABA-receptor complexes at binding domains located close to or allosterically coupled to benzodiazepine receptors."

Eszopiclone is similar in action, use, warnings, etc. to zolpidem and zaleplon.

There have been multiple reports for all the three previous sleeping medications of patients sleep walking, sleep driving, sleep cooking, sleep eating, sleep sexing, etc. Caution should be exercised to make sure that the patient uses the least effective dose of these medications, for the shortest duration of need, with specific review of physiological and psychological comorbidities (including addiction matters), with frequent review of therapy, and with safeguards in place to keep the patient who takes these medications safe.

This next drug is a sleeper, but is not a benzodiazepine, at all!

Ramelteon (Rozerem): This medication has a different chemical "chassis", and a different mechanism of action from the benzodiazepines. It is included in this part of the book solely because of the use of Rozerem to induce sleep.

How does ramelteon (Rozerem) work? This drug is a **_melatonin agonist_**, having **NO** effect on any of the following neurotransmitters:

- ✓ GABA
- ✓ Serotonin
- ✓ Acetylcholine
- ✓ Dopamine
- ✓ Norepinephrine
- ✓ Opiate receptors

This drug should not be used in patients with severe liver problems, or patients taking fluvoxamine (Luvox) as the fluvoxamine increases the level of ramelteon 190 fold! Ramelteon may decrease testosterone levels and cause an increase in prolactin levels. Ramelteon should not be used in people with severe sleep apnea or COPD due to a possibility of angioedema involving the tongue, glottis or larynx, and should not be taken with or after a fatty meal, or with alcohol.

And now a "sister" to that sleeper, used for a really interesting condition

Tasimelteon (Hetlioz) - This is a brand-new (well, approved in 2014) melatonin agonist that is approved by the FDA for "non-24 hour sleep-wake disorder" in totally blind individuals. It is mentioned here in this book because like ramelteon (Rozerem) - note the similarities of the generic name! - this, too, has some chemical similarities with ramelteon.

Some drugs of abuse: date rape medications

There is a need to discuss at length two other medications, one classified as an antianxiety treatment, and the other, well, not classified.

Flunitrazepam (Rohypnol, not marketed in the U.S.):
This is included under the "antianxiety" medications solely due to the fact that this is also a benzodiazepine.

This has a street name of "Roophie" and is a date-rape drug. This BZD is a sedative/hypnotic, and is used as an intoxicant.

Yes, this is available over the internet.

Flunitrazepam is similar in chemical structure and action to triazolam (Halcion) (a "sleeper" mentioned earlier in this book.) Understand, however, that any combination of a sufficient amount of a benzodiazepine and alcohol could produce a similar effect to flunitrazepam (Rohypnol.)

Gamma hydroxybutyrate (GHB)[37]:
Have you yet heard of GHB, gentle reader? While not a benzodiazepine, and not used (or approved) as a treatment for anxiety, it follows Rohypnol in that this, too, is a date-rape drug. GHB, like the benzodiazepine medications, has significant effect on GABA. For this reason, GHB is mentioned in this book at this time during the discussion of Rohypnol and the relationship between GABA and GHB. Then, the text will again take up the discussion of the other anxiolytic medications.

GHB use is increasing, and there are reports of Rohypnol use decreasing (although this may vary, depending on where the reader lives and works.) GHB was once limited to large warehouse scenes such as "raves," but GHB is now a party drug.

GHB has been grouped with, and confused with, other drugs in the "date-rape drug" category such as flunitrazepam (Rohypnol.) GHB, like flunitrazepam (Rohypnol), can be slipped easily into a drink and given to an unsuspecting victim, who often does not remember being assaulted. GHB, when used with alcohol is especially dangerous.

Possible symptoms of GHB use-
It may give the user a feeling of euphoria, that "Everything is fine."
What was it used for?
GHB was first developed for use as a general anæsthetic; GHB did not work very well to prevent pain, so its use as an anesthetic declined. And GHB became a drug of abuse.

---

[37] Street names for GHB include: "Georgia Home Boy", "Liquid E", "Liquid X", "Juice", "Mils", "Liquid G", and "Fantasy."

The observation that GHB may cause the release of growth hormone led some people, especially athletes and body-builders, to take this chemical because they thought GHB would increase muscle development; this is how GHB got "into" the drug culture.

At the time body builders were using GHB, GHB was available as a dietary supplement and as such was not regulated by the US Food and Drug Administration.

GHB is similar in activity to alcohol, in that GHB is a central nervous system depressant; GHB takes only minutes to make a user lose control, forget what is happening, or lose consciousness.

And that is why GHB is used as a rape drug.

GHB is colorless, odorless, and has a slightly salty taste. Scary, and surprising, the synthetic form of

GHB contains some of the same ingredients as floor stripper and industrial cleaners! That adds to the problem of GHB being used as a date-rape drug, as GHB is really easy to make, and it does not leave tell-tale "markers" like the benzodiazepine medications listed above. Yes, there are blood and urine tests for the use of benzodiazepines, but not for GHB, because GHB is found naturally in the human body.

Equipotent doses of GHB can have different effects in different people- a dose that makes one person feel euphoric might cause another person to become quite ill.

GHB can be lethal, and addictive; the US Drug Enforcement Agency was able to link GHB to 58 deaths since 1990, with 5,700 overdoses have been recorded just up until 2005 (Kurwana, 2005). There are reports that suggest GHB can cause dependence (Brunt, Koeter, Hertoghs, van Noorden, & van den Brink, 2013).

Detection of the drug is hard, as GHB is present in mammalian tissue, a neurotransmitter normally found in the brain (Schröck, Hari, König, Auwärter, Schürch, & Weinmann, 2013)! Because ER doctors have difficulty in detecting GHB they often have problems treating overdose.

Unfortunately, GHB can also be manufactured synthetically in a lab.

How GHB works in the brain:

GHB is produced normally in the brain through the synthesis of GABA, with some of the greatest concentrations of GHB found in the thalamus, the hypothalamus, as well as in the *substantia nigra*. Indeed, GHB affects several neurotransmitters in the brain. For example, dopamine activity decrease is seen especially in the basal ganglia, and is probably the result of the inhibition of the release of dopamine from synaptic terminals. GHB can activate GHB receptors and GABA receptors on neurons in the brain.

In 1990, after numerous reports that GHB caused illness, the FDA began investigating the drug, and GHB is now classified as an illegal substance in the United States. It is still used overseas.

A derivative of GHB, **sodium oxybate (Xyrem)**, is FDA approved as of 11/26/2005 to treat cataplexy in narcolepsy and excessive daytime sleepiness in narcolepsy.

Turning back to the anxiolytic class of psychotropic medications, the next category of anxiolytics will include:

Antihistamines   **β-blockers**   **Azapirone**

All these drugs have one major component in common that separates them from the BZDs (other than chemical structure): There is little, if any, physiological dependence. By the same token, these may not be as effective in some patients (especially those who have had previous therapy with BZDs). Also, these medications are thought to affect neurotransmitters other than GABA.

Next anxiolytic "class"- the antihistamines:

Antihistamines are thought to "work" by decreasing the effect of the neurotransmitter histamine. That means that these medications are histamine antagonists- or are antagonistic to histamine- or are "anti-"histamine. Get it?

Diphenhydramine (Benadryl)

Classification: Sedative, antihistamine.
Used as: Somnotic, anxiolytic.

Diphenhydramine is a very weak anxiolytic, but may be useful with children or when other agents are contraindicated. Interesting, this medication has has been used with similar results to benztropine for extrapyramidal symptoms (EPS) caused by antipsychotic use.

This medication is not bad for short-term (less than 7 days) use without a prescription- and is the active ingredient in the over-the-counter sleeping agents Sominex, Nytol, and ZzzQuil. There has been research that patients using diphenhydramine report "improved state of sleep" with no significant effects on "interruption of sleep", "feelings on awakening", or "severity of insomnia." (Kudo & Kithara, 1990) It seemed that patients naïve to diphenhydramine had significantly better therapeutic response in the Kudo study.

Diphenhydramine is much less expensive than most sedative-hypnotics, but does have some anticholinergic side effects (dry mouth, dry eyes, constipation, urinary retention, etc.) and does have an effect on the respiratory tract (dries up secretions.) Allergies to this drug are rare, and when compared to barbiturates or benzodiazepines, overdose easily managed.

Diphenhydramine is rarely abused, and withdrawal is not usually a problem for most patients. Additionally, diphenhydramine is relatively less likely to induce tolerance and dependence.

Hydroxyzine (Vistaril, Atarax[38])

Classification: Sedative, antihistamine.
Used as: Anxiolytic.

Hydroxyzine is used to treat anxiety and tension associated with psychoneurosis, as well as being used as an adjunct to organic disease states that may manifest in anxiety states. Hydroxyzine is used as a premedication for dental and surgical procedures, in "acute emotional problems" as well as in

---

[38] Atarax is usually encountered in dermatology, and is used to treat various types of conditions where itchiness is significant. Atarax and Vistaril are both hydroxyzine salts: Atarax is "hydroxyzine hydrochloride" while Vistaril is "hydroxyzine pamoate." To understand what "salts" are in chemistry, understand that when one mixes an acid with a base one gets a salt as the yield. As example, when mixing sodium (a base) with chloride (an acid) one gets sodium chloride- table salt. But mixing potassium (a base) with chloride yields potassium chloride. Both are "salts" of chloride.

treating the client with alcoholism (to deter anxious states due to the alcohol withdrawal) including treating *delirium tremens* (the DTs.)

Hydroxyzine has some benefits for helping treat allergic conditions with "strong emotional overlay"- like pruritus or chronic urticaria. One may have heard of a "nervous rash."

Of note is that hydroxyzine may be of significant help to cardiac patients to allay the associated anxiety and apprehension experienced by those patients.

Hydroxyzine is used as a sedative, and may be used as a premedication and also following general anæsthesia, and may be beneficial (delivered via intramuscular injection) to treat post-partum anxiety and nausea. For pain patients, it seems that when hydroxyzine is coadministered with narcotic analgesics, there can be a reduction of the narcotic dose. Hydroxyzine is not bad for an itch, either. As example, another form of this drug is known by the brand name of Atarax, and Atarax is used for rashes and in dermatology. (See footnote on the previous page.)

Hydroxyzine is a weak anxiolytic that may be used when other agents are contraindicated, like, for instance, with a patient having an anxiety attack who also has a history of substance abuse. This drug affects pretty much the whole of the brain, including the limbic system and brainstem reticular formation. Hydroxyzine is much less expensive than most sedative-hypnotics, and, like diphenhydramine (Benadryl- discussed in the previous section of this book) has some anticholinergic side effects – that dry mouth, dry eye, etc., problem- and like diphenhydramine does have a "drying of the mucous" effect on the respiratory tract.

Hydroxyzine is one of the more "interesting" drugs in that it is chemically related to chlorpromazine (Thorazine.) That is not the "interesting part"[39]- indeed, the "interesting part" of this is that in 1950 chlorpromazine (Thorazine) as developed and marketed as an antihistamine! Indeed, in 1950, if you, gentle reader, had poison ivy you might be given Thorazine.

And you would not itch!

...might not "do" much of anything...

Hydroxyzine is metabolized (using enzymes!) into cetirizine (Zyrtec- the over-the-counter [OTC] antihistamine!) in the liver (as well as to other metabolites.)

Hydroxyzine should not be given to pregnant or nursing mothers, and, just like diphenhydramine (Benadryl), allergies to this drug are rare. Also, just like diphenhydramine, hydroxyzine overdose is easily managed, and hydroxyzine is rarely abused. Good news! Withdrawal from hydroxyzine is not usually a problem, and hydroxyzine is relatively less likely to induce tolerance and dependence.

---

[39] See the discussion of how the antipsychotic medications like chlorpromazine (Thorazine) were developed from quinine and methylene blue on pages 13 and 14 of this book!

There are other antihistamines which could theoretically be used to treat anxiety states, but diphenhydramine and hydroxyzine are the two most often encountered when treating mental health patients.[40]

---

[40] Here are some other antihistamines. Remember, the mechanism of action includes blocking the histamine H^1 receptors. Note also the names "loratadine" and "desloratadine" as well as "cetirizine" and "levocetirizine." These are isomeric relatives one to the other, and this concept will be explained more fully later in this book.

Antihistamine	Common name
Chlorpheniramine	Chlor-Trimeton
Meclizine	Antivert; Bonine; Dramamine
Promethazine	Phenergan
Cetirizine	Zyrtec (see above- an active metabolite of hydroxyzine!)
Desloratadine	Clarinex
Loratadine	Claritin
Fexofenadine	Allegra
Levocetirizine	Xyral

Now, the ß-blockers

These are best described as being "beta-adrenergic blockers" but the shortened phrase is almost always used to describe these medications. These medications are thought to have an effect on reducing norepinephrine activity, effectively reducing the "flight" part of the "fight or flight response."

In this class, there are a quite few "members.[41]" All have extremely similar functions, so this book will describe only the prototype:

Propranolol (Inderal)
Classification: Adrenergic blocking agent.
Used as: Anxiolytic (as well as a bunch of other things.)

ß-blockers might be much better for clients with prominent cardiovascular symptoms of anxiety (remember the saber toothed tiger and the "fight or flight response" discussed earlier in this book.) these medications have been shown to be effective for "essential tremor" in some patients. Side effects would include the "beta blocker blues"- a clinical depression (see the footnote below.)

The ß-blocker medications are much less effective than BZDs, generally, at easing anxiety states, and the ß-blockers do have an effect on the respiratory tract (again, see the footnote below). The ß-blocker medications are relatively safe to use, and overdose is easily managed- just maintain the heart rate, breathing, blood sugar, and blood pressure. This class of antianxiety medications is rarely abused, but withdrawal must be done carefully for physiological as well as psychological reasons.[42] The ß-blocker class of

---

[41] Here is a rather comprehensive list of the ß-blockers currently available in the United States as of the writing of this book. Note carefully- these all have the same suffix: "-olol." This is how one may deduce that a medication is a member of the ß-blocker class. If the generic name of the drug ends "-olol" that drug is a ß-blocker.

Carteolol (used in ophthalmology)	Labetolol	Nadolol
Penbutolol	Pindolol	Propranolol
Sotalol (note minor change in suffix)	Timolol (oral use plus ophthalmology)	Acebutolol
Atenolol	Betaxolol	Bisoprolol
Esmolol (injection only)	Metoprolol	Nebivolol
These have different clinical applications, but all share some of the mechanism of action.		

[42] Also reflect, though, that if one gives a ß-blocker for ANY reason, and these medications are used for everything from high blood pressure to anxiety to controlling heart rhythms to PTSD and migraine headaches- that some possible side effect may be noted. Specifically, low blood pressure (even if the medication is taken for another reason) which might increase having the patient fall over upon arising. Patients with asthma and chronic bronchitis should be careful with these medications. ß-blockers can affect blood sugar metabolism, and can cause clinical depression as a side effect. Also reflect that if a patient has been taking a ß-blocker- again for any reason- and then suddenly stops taking the medication that the patient may then experience some of the symptoms listed above- like a rapid heart rate. The patient may think that this "rapid heart rate" is anxiety, or even a panic attack. For this reason, any patient who has his or her ß-blocker dose reduced or even discontinued should be monitored for symptoms of anxiety.

antianxiety medications is relatively less likely to induce tolerance and dependence.

Only one Azapirone will be presented-

Buspirone (BuSpar)

Classification: Azapirone, a selective $5HT_{1A}$ agonist- yes, an antianxiety drug that does not "work" on dopamine or norepinephrine.

Used as: Anxiolytic.

With the use of buspirone drowsiness is not a problem, generally. This medication may take 5 to 7 days to work, and optimal therapeutic results are generally seen after 3 to 4 weeks of treatment. Alcohol does not potentiate the antianxiety effect, which may be an issue with the benzodiazepines (BZDs) and the barbiturates. The exact action of buspirone is unknown, just like the fact that the exact action of ANY medication is truly unknown.

Buspirone is not chemically related to BZDs, barbiturates, sedatives, or other anxiolytics; and it is for this reason that buspirone may be the source of therapy failure in clients previously treated with BZDs (but there are no established studies to support this). The reason that some patient may fail with buspirone is that the patient does not "feel" the drug "kicking in." Compare this to the patient who can tell you exactly when the Xanax (alprazolam) begins to work.

The use of buspirone with haloperidol (Haldol) may increase haloperidol levels. Another possible drug interaction of note is that buspirone may cause mania if co-administered with disulfiram (Antabuse), a medication sometimes, but rarely, still used to treat alcoholism. The combination of clomipramine (a tricyclic antidepressant known by the brand name as Anafranil) and buspirone may cause hypertension and anxiety.

Buspirone may be said to be safer to use than other antianxiety medications, as overdose easily managed (again, just do supportive physiological and psychological care), this medication is rarely abused, and as a rule withdrawal not a problem (as opposed to the potential seizure issues with BZD withdrawal, cardiac and psychological concerns with the β-blocker withdrawal, and possible death if someone tried to stop barbiturates.) Buspirone is relatively less likely to induce tolerance and dependence. Safety and efficacy has not been established in children younger than 18, and elderly folks appear to not have any problem with this medication, unless there is severe hepatic or renal impairment.

Do remember, this is a serotonin drug, so serotonin syndrome should always be considered, especially when a patient is taking other serotonin medications.

Now for the mood stabilizers

Several of these drugs have been traditionally used for control of seizure activity. It is not uncommon, however, for drugs in this class to be used for "mood stabilization." Following the theme of this book, not all the medications used for mood stabilization will be discussed in this instant chapter. Candidly, the mechanism of action, side effects, etc., do not vary that much from one drug in this class to another, and theoretically any of the antiseizure medications might be used to treat bipolar disorders. For information, though, here is a list of the common medications used as "mood stabilizers", but theoretically any of the medications used for treatment of seizures could be used to treat bipolar disorder, specifically the symptoms of mania and hypomania.

Here is the list of common medications used to treat bipolar disorder:

CARBAMAZEPINE	DIVALPROEX · LAMOTRIGINE	VALPROIC ACID	LITHIUM

There are other anticonvulsant medications, too. The table below is presented in this section ONLY due to the facts that these medications may have a similar mechanism of action to the drugs detailed elsewhere in this text. The anticonvulsant medications may therefore affect clinical mood presentations, and may have similar side effects and warnings, regardless of clinical use. Also note that many of these medications have "gab" in the generic names- deference to "GABA." Note that some of these have significant warnings, often when used in children. Again, these are NOT normally used to treat bipolar disorders.

Clobazam	Ethosuximide	Ezo**gab**ine	Felbamate
Fosphenytoin sodium	Lacosamide	Oxcarbazepine	Phenytoin
Primidone	Rufinamide	Vi**gaba**trin	Zonisamide

Note that the antipsychotic medications also used to treat bipolar disorders are not listed on this chart above, nor are the antidepressant medications. The antipsychotic medications and antidepressants will be discussed elsewhere in this book.

How do these "mood stabilizers" work?

Well, no one knows for sure![43]

---

[43] An argument could be made that the precise mechanism of action of **ANY** drug used in treating mental health conditions is not precisely known. Remember: medications are given to patients not because of the mechanism of action, but rather because the medications result in a change in the patients' clinical presentation. See page 9 and the discussion of infection and mental illness.

All the anticonvulsants routinely used to treat bipolar disorder are believed to reduce the release of monoamine neurotransmitters, like dopamine (the "fight" of the fight or flight response); norepinephrine (the "flight" of the fight or flight response); serotonin; epinephrine; etc.

It is for this concept that these medications are thought to decrease the activity of these neurotransmitters that the effect must be somehow related to increasing GABA activity in a manner similar to how the barbiturates and benzodiazepines "work." The reader will remember the discussion of the "brakes of the brain" found in this book on page 39. The mood stabilizers are also thought to be blockers of voltage-gated sodium channels (reflect back to the previous discussion of "short-circuiting of the cells") as well as possibly affecting the glutamate system in the brain.

Remember- look at what the body does normally, and either increase that response with an agonist or decrease that response with an antagonist. If the body uses glutamate as an excitatory neurotransmitter, then a drug may be used that could theoretically reduce that glutamate excitation. In this case, that reduction of excitation is due to increasing the inhibitory effect of GABA on all sorts of neurotransmitters.

Lithium is a little odd. This drug is not thought to have an effect on GABA, but rather is suspected to work at various points on the neuron between the nucleus and the synapse. While the exact mechanism of action of lithium remains unknown, some of how lithium acts in the body is thought to be inhibition of an enzyme known as GSK-3b (ah, remember the discussion of enzymes also on page 23!)

By inhibiting the action of this enzyme, it is thought that there is an effect relieving pressure on the circadian clock - which is believed to be often malfunctioning in people with bipolar disorder.

Further, lithium may positively modulate gene transcription of Brain Derived Neurotrophic Factor (BDNF), which may result in seeing an increase in neural plasticity and possibly explain some of the therapeutic effects of lithium. Lithium may also increase the synthesis of serotonin, and may also "short-circuit" the electrical transmission in the axon.

Valproic acid (and valproate), carbamazepine and oxcarbazepine (brand name Trileptal, this drug is not presented in this book other than at this moment; oxcarbazepine is a "sister" to carbamazepine) may provide the mood-stabilizing effects as a result of affecting the GABAergic system (the "brakes of the brain"); lamotrigine (Lamictal) is known to decrease the patient's cortisol response to stress- taking the hormonal part of the "fight" and the "flight" down a notch.

There may even be some involvement in affecting the arachidonic acid cascade by lithium, carbamazepine, and even valproate. Something to consider is that one possible downstream target of several mood stabilizers such as lithium, valproate, and carbamazepine is the arachidonic acid cascade- and this may be why patients in chronic pain are also often prescribed these medications. (Rao, Lee, Rapoport, & Brazinet, 2008)

There are some concerns about "mood stabilizers"....

On March of 2005 the FDA requested the 14 manufacturers of these drugs provide safety information relating to an increase in suicide. Of note: This list of manufacturers includes the pharmacy companies that make Neurontin, Topamax, and Lamictal.

This is an outgrowth of some legal actions, notably the work of New York attorney Lawrence Finklestein, who in May 2004 filed a Citizen's Petition with the FDA asking for there to be a "BLACK BOX WARNING" for these drugs. Attorney Finklestein submitted 271 "adverse event" reports to the FDA detailing successful suicide attempts by patients taking Neurontin. (Pringle, 2007)

This book will not address ALL the anticonvulsants that are used as "mood stabilizers"

Just selected ones...and the reason is that many of them are "me-too" drugs. This means: "I am a mood stabilizer!" "Me, too!"

This book will include the antimanic drug lithium.
One cannot forget that some of the atypical antipsychotics like Risperdal and Seroquel and Abilify are used as "mood stabilizers", too- but those medications will be discussed in another section of this book.

To reiterate: anticonvulsants, as a "rule", inhibit neuronal firing; many times the proposed mechanism of action is, indeed, stimulation of GABA. Sometimes the proposed mechanism of action has to do with "short-circuiting" the cells, by way of inhibition of either sodium or chloride ion channels. Remember the barbiturates and the benzodiazepines? See the similarities?

Carbamazepine (Tegretol[44], Epitol[32], Carbatrol[32], and Equetro)

Classification: Iminostilbene[45]; reduces synaptic transmission within the trigeminal nucleus (for *tic douloureux*); reduces posttetanic potentiation of synaptic transmission.

Used as: Anticonvulsant; to treat trigeminal neuralgia, and, in January 2005, Equetro was approved by the FDA to treat...Bipolar Disorder.[46]

Non-approved uses for carbamazepine:

- Schizoaffective disorder
- Resistant schizophrenia
- Dyscontrol syndrome
- Associated with limbic system dysfunction
- Intermittent explosive disorder
- PTSD
- Atypical psychosis
- Management of withdrawal from either/or Alcohol, Cocaine, Benzodiazepines
- Restless legs syndrome
- Painful neuromas
- Sedative
- Antiarrhythmic
- Antidiuretic
- Muscle relaxant
- Analgesic (nonneuritic pain syndromes)
- Painful neuromas
- Phantom limb pain
- Chorea in children
- Neurogenic or central diabetes insipidus

---

[44] Tegretol, Carbatrol, and Epitol are not FDA approved to treat bipolar disorder- only Equetro is. That does not mean that these two medications may not be used to treat the condition, just that these drugs lack the official approval.

[45] Remember from the discussion of "where these drugs come from" on page 13 (in footnote)- the "chassis" for carbamazepine is imminodibenzyl or "Summer Blue"- the same "chassis" from which Tofranil comes. (Healy).

[46] The FDA pounded on Equetro for having incorrect information listed in the Professional Circular on June 25, 2012. The manufacturer of Equetro did not list warnings about the use of this drug in pregnancy, in patients with seizure disorder or increased intraocular pressure; that there is a possible activation of a latent psychosis, and, in elderly patients that confusion or agitation may occur. The manufacturer also did not mention a warning about the use of Equetro with a specific AIDS medication (delavirdine). The manufacturer did list issues about increased suicidal thoughts or behavior, but did not include the phrase: "[a]nyone considering prescribing Equetro or any other AED (antiepileptic drug) must balance the risk of suicidal thought or behavior with the risk of untreated illness" and that "patients, their caregivers, and families should be informed that AEDs increase the risk of suicidal thoughts and behaviors and should be advised of the need to be alert for the emergence or worsening of the signs and symptoms of depression, any unusual changes in mood or behavior, or the emergence of suicidal thoughts, behavior, or thoughts about self-harm." The FDA was also concerned that the Professional insert- and the Equetro webpages, incorrectly stated that AEDs "may increase" the risk of suicidal thoughts or behavior when, in fact, the PI indicated that a direct relationship between AEDs and suicidal behavior and ideation has been determined.

Last, the FDA had concerns that the Equetro webpage had "unsubstantiated claims" including that Equetro would relieve acute manic and mixed symptoms of bipolar I Disorders...**Without Inducing Weight Gain** (emphasis added by the FDA.) Additionally, the FDA had concerns that this unsubstantiated and misleading quote appeared in the webpage for Equetro: **"The HAM-D SCALE reveals that Bipolar I Patients treated with Equetro (carbamazepine) Extended-Release Capsules showed no worsening of depression** (again, emphasis by the FDA) (Department of Health & Human Services, Food and Drug Administration, 2012)."

Drug comparisons:

It is hard to have a comparison between carbamazepine and other mood stabilizers, as the comparison must be with antiepileptic agents like phenobarbital, phenytoin, and primidone.

Carbamazepine may be used for clients who are either unresponsive or intolerant to valproate and/or lithium; in these cases, carbamazepine is not a bad choice of agent.

Drug interactions and other concerns would include quite a few drug-drug interactions; possible dyscrasias. There is a significant risk of aplastic anæmia and agranulocytosis with this drug (5 to 8 times greater than normally seen in the general population).[47]

Carbamazepine is an enzyme-inducer- which means that this medication may cause other medications to be "eaten up" by enzymes quicker (which, theoretically, could result in a decreased effectiveness of the "other" drugs.)

Carbamazepine may not be a bad adjunctive choice for refractory bipolar disorder, and may work better than lithium in clients with mixed bipolar conditions or with rapid cyclers.

There is a need for more in-depth studies that might be helpful in confirming both short- and long-term effectiveness for the treatment of bipolar disorder with carbamazepine.

Valproic acid (Depakene, Stavzor) and derivatives valproate sodium (Depacon) divalproex sodium (Depakote, Depakote CP, and Depakote ER)[48]

Classification: Carboxylic acid derivatives; may work by suppressing repetitive neuronal firing through inhibition of voltage-sensitive sodium channel.[49]

Incidentally, there are some other proposed modes of action, in that the derivatives of valproic acid might increase concentrations of γ-aminobutyric acid (GABA) in the brain. That should sound familiar: "the brakes of the brain!" Remember that GABA is an inhibitory neurotransmitter in the CNS. With divalproate, there are yet other proposed modes of action, in that this drug may also inhibit the enzymes that catabolize GABA or may block the reuptake of GABA into nerve endings and the glial cells (rather like a "GABA reuptake inhibitor" or "GABA receptor blocker").

Official FDA approvals:

For divalproate: (Depakene) include treatment of epilepsy and in migraine prevention; for valproic acid (Stavzor and Depakote ER) both are

---

[47] This information comes from the FDA New Drug Application for Carbatrol. See: www.fda.gov/downloards/Drugs/Drug SafetyNewsletter/UCM148014.pdf, page 3.)

[48] For this medication, the author will call all of these medications "divalproate." While there are indeed chemical differences between these various products, all are thought to have similar mechanism of action.

[49] Sounds like "short circuiting the cells", does it not?

approved to treat mania, epilepsy, and to prevent migraine; for valproate sodium (Depacon) only epilepsy.

Used as:

Anticonvulsant	Antimanic	Antimigraine

Drug comparisons:

Divalproate is used for mania as well as bipolar disorder. Divalproate may be better tolerated by some clients than lithium, and may work better in rapid cyclers and mixed mania clients (but the jury is still out on this).

There are concerns about using divalproate, other than those listed above for all the AEDs- there are quite a few drug-drug interactions, and this medication seems to have a higher risk for patients of successful suicide and suicide attempts than does lithium. Liver toxicity, pancreatitis, and major congenital malformations have resulted in a Black Box Warning for these medications entitled: "WARNING: LIFE-THREATENING ADVERSE REACTIONS."

A very troubling article was published in 2013 that suggests that the use of divalproate might cause an increase in the number of children being born who will receive a diagnosis of autism (Christensen, Grønborg, Sørensen, Schendel, Parner, Pedersen, & Vestergaard, 2003).

Other non-approved uses:

Divalproate may be helpful in treating agitation or explosive temper that is comorbid with ADHD. This ought to make sense, as this puts "the brakes on the brain". Divalproate is also used to treat singultus- chronic and unremitting hiccough, a condition that has also been successfully treated with the phenothiazine tranquilizers like Thorazine.

Divalproate has been useful in select populations (clients with dementia, elderly folk) to help control aggressive behaviors/agitated states- but remember the warnings with antiepileptic drugs (AEDs) and elderly patients who are confused (see footnote on the bottom of page 64.)

Gabapentin (Neurontin, Horizant[50], Gralise[51], Fanatrex[52], Gabarone[38])
Classification: Anticonvulsant; this medication is a derivative of GABA.

Gabapentin does not show affinity for receptor binding or reuptake blockade at the "normal" or "expected" sites; rat studies show binding sites in the hippocampus and neocortex.

Used as: Anticonvulsant; treatment of postherpetic neuralgia (shingles) in adults

---

[50] Horizant is gabapentin enacarbil, a derivative of gabapentin, and is FDA approved to treat restless legs syndrome and postherpetic neuralgia (shingles.).

[51] Gralise is gabapentin, but is FDA approved only for treatment of shingles pain.

[52] Gabarone and Fanatrex suspension has been approved to treat nerve pain after herpes, and as an additional medication to treat partial seizures.

Unofficial uses of gabapentin include:

℞	Treatment for bipolar disorders
℞	Treatment of tremors associated with multiple sclerosis (MS)
℞	Antianxiety agent
℞	Analgesic
℞	Specifically, to treat neuropathic pain
℞	Migraine prophylaxis
℞	Control of substance abuse

Drug comparisons:

With the successes of valproate and carbamazepine in treating seizure disorders, this drug is being investigated, is and has been used for "non-epileptiform" therapeutic uses. Gabapentin (Neurontin) seems to have some benefits over other medications in this class, notably that there is no need for therapeutic drug monitoring. Additionally, there are minimal drug interactions and this drug has a favorable side effect profile.

More drug comparisons:

Gabapentin has been reported to provide benefit during alcohol withdrawal (there is quite a bit of research on this for almost two decades) (Myrick, Malcolm, & Brady, 1998; Muncie, Yasinian, & Ogé, 2013). This medication has been shown to benefit clients who have agitation as a presentation of dementia (but one has to be careful using this with elderly clients who may be more sensitive to the effects of this medication.)

Of note is that there is a decrease in bioavailability of gabapentin as the dose increases. What this means is that there is a "ceiling effect" in that after a certain (patient-specific) dose, there is limited benefit seen in increasing the dose. Understand that there may be some concerns about dosage adjustments and bioavailability, as published, well-designed studies on efficacy are lacking. Additionally, there is limited information on the use of gabapentin as an adjunctive agent with other mood stabilizers.

In children who have epilepsy (age 3 to 12) there have been some problems, including emotional lability, which is primarily presented as behavioral problems (6% vs. 1.3% for placebo.) These behavioral problems present as symptoms that sound vaguely like ADHD!

- ℞ Hostility, including aggression (5.2% vs. 1.3% for placebo);
- ℞ Thought disorder, including concentration problems and change in school performance (1.7% vs. 0% for placebo);
- ℞ Hyperkineses, including restlessness and hyperactivity (4.7% vs. 2.9%.)

Here are some ethical and practical questions about gabapentin:

Understand that as recently as the year 2005, 90% of gabapentin (Neurontin) sales were for "off-label" diagnoses; the manufacturer is marketing BOTH a higher-priced "Brand Name" (Neurontin) as well as a lesser-priced "Generic Equivalent" (gabapentin.)

"How does that make you feel?"
"What does the manufacturer think about this?"
Here are some other medications that are primarily used to treat seizures, but which may also have benefit for bipolar disorders (as well as other conditions listed.)

Tiagabine (Gabitril)

An interesting drug, the manufacturer says this is a "GABA reuptake inhibitor," which would mean that the use of this drug increases the amount of GABA in the synaptic space. Once again, increasing GABA (theoretically) results in a decrease in 33% of all CNS activity.

This medication is indeed FDA approved to be used as an adjunctive therapy for partial seizures in adults and children at least 12 years of age, but is being investigated for treatment of bipolar disorders, PTSD in adults, and refractory seizures in children. (Spratto & Woods, 2013)

Levetiracetam (Keppra)

This drug is approved as adjunctive therapy for children as young as age 4, as well as adults, who have various types of seizure activity. Clinicians see levetiracetam being used in patients in neuroscience departments of hospitals quite frequently.

This medication is being investigated for use in prevention of migraines in adults, adolescents, and children; to treat bipolar disorder in adults and children; and, interestingly enough, also for treatment of tardive dyskinesia (TD) caused by the use of other neuroleptic medications, like the antipsychotic medications. That last aspect is significant, but also significant in that this medication does not PREVENT the occurrence of TD, but is being studied for treatment of TD[53] (Spratto).

The levetiracetam (Keppra) mode of action- well, that is unknown. This looks like it may work in the hippocampus (remember, traumatic memory seems to be consolidated in the hippocampus), seeming to "lower kindling"- a term coming from neurology to explain the subsyndromal status found in clients with epileptiform disorders. "Kindling?" What this means is that levetiracetam may act in the CNS synaptic membranes to "prevent hypersynchronization of epileptiform burst firing and propagation of seizure activity without affecting normal neuronal excitability" (Spratto)." Nah, "kindling" is easier to say.

Levetiracetam (Keppra) action has been shown to "oppose the activity of negative modulators of GABA- and glycine-gated currents in neuronal cell culture" (Surges, Volynski, and Walker, 2008); guess that means if one opposes negative modulators one then sees positive modulation. As mentioned above, the mechanism of action is unknown.

---

[53] Tardive dyskinesia will be discussed later in this book in the chapter dealing with antipsychotic medications. Know that TD has been known to occur with other classes of medication, too.

Topiramate (Topamax)

Classification: Monosaccharide; topiramate is not related structurally to other agents in this class.

Used as: Anticonvulsant; to prevent migraine; investigationally as a mood stabilizer.

A serious drug interaction notice from the FDA was issued in January 2006 about topiramate when used with valproate

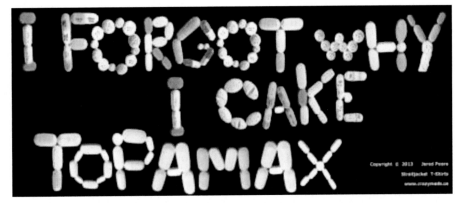

Used with the gracious permission of Jerod Poore, 2014b

(Depakote) - some patients developed hyperammonemia and encephalopathy associated with concomitant Depakote use (Noh, Kim, Chu, Jung, Moon, & Lee, 2013). Additionally, FDA now requires a warning about an increase in the occurrence of neonatal cleft palate when this is used by the mother during pregnancy (U.S. Food and Drug Administration, 2011; Janssen Pharmaceuticals, Inc., 2012).

More on topiramate (Topamax):

This medication is thought to increase the frequency at which GABA activates GABA receptors, which means that this drug potentiates the activity of the inhibitory transmitter. Also, action potentials are blocked (that old "short-circuit thingy".) Topiramate (Topamax) has an elimination half-life of 21 hours, which is why this medication could be prescribed once a day (for migraines; for seizure control this is usually dosed twice daily.) This medication has an odd warning, in that if may cause oligohidrosis (decreased perspiration) which could result in hyperthermia.

This drug may interact with phenytoin (Dilantin) and carbamazepine (Tegretol, Carbatrol, and others), and, as an anti-seizure medication, covers the same anticonvulsant spectra as does carbamazepine and phenytoin.

Topiramate (Topamax) is also used off-label for weight reduction, which may be caused by the concomitant use of various psychotropic agents, such as some of the antidepressants, the antipsychotics, and various other drugs. Note that the FDA-approved weight loss medication Qsymia contains topiramate and phentermine (and phentermine was one-half of the combination "fen-phen" which caused some patients to develop fatal primary pulmonary hypertension.)

Lithium (Eskalith, Cibalith-S)

Classification: Metal, a mineral salt.

Lithium alters cation transport in nerve and muscle cells (cations are "negative ions") –all this means is that lithium "short-circuits the cells."
Lithium blocks the release of thyroid hormones T_3 and T_4. Note once again that

hormones and neurotransmitters are intimately related. Also reflect that a patient who has **hyper**thyroidism (high thyroid function) may have a manic clinical presentation, while a patient with **hypo**thyroidism (low thyroid function) may appear to have symptoms of depression. Once again: look at what the body does "normally" then either increase or decrease that normal function. This also speaks to the fact that decreasing thyroid functioning- due to the blocking of the release of thyroid hormone- might result in side effects of depression and lethargy. This also explains why some patients who take lithium may develop goiters. Lithium may have some effect on blood cell forming (hematopoiesis), and may produce neutrophilia.

Lithium affects catecholamine metabolism- and several catecholamines have been discussed as the basis for psychopharmacology in this book: dopamine, serotonin, norepinephrine, adrenaline, etc.

Used as:

- Antidepressant therapy adjunct
- Antimanic
  - Granulopoietic
- Vascular headache prophylactic
- Prophylaxis of bipolar disorder

Drug comparisons:

Lithium is the "first-line" treatment of bipolar illness, even though valproate and carbamazepine are frequently used now.

There are quite a few side effects with lithium. The most notable is that the LD_{50} (lethal dose) is rather close to the ED_{50} (effective dose). This is why lithium blood levels are so important. Additionally, hydration is a must. It is not uncommon to see patients who take lithium successfully and then become toxic because they perspire and do not rehydrate, like in hot summer months during exercise or cold months during snow sports like skiing.

Some comments about lithium for bipolar disorder- this is a good choice for clients who have ongoing substance abuse problems (because this will not be "abused"), who have atypical mania, who are rapid cyclers, or who have mixed bipolar states.

On to the antidepressants!

Ah, more brain neurotransmitter discussion! The current theoretical underpinnings of the cause of depression would be serotonin, norepinephrine, and dopamine "dysregulation." Remember the previous discussions in this book about:

1. People being chased by a saber-toothed tiger are not depressed (norepinephrine- the "flight" of the flight-or-flight response);
2. Giving a medication that mimics that response could then be used to treat depression (the tricyclic antidepressants are thought to "work" on norepinephrine- the "tiger chemical");
3. Tricyclic antidepressants may have side effects like cardiac dysrhythmias, and norepinephrine affects the heart rate;
4. The exact mechanism of action of antidepressants is not known. Drugs are given to patients, and if those patients feel better, then those drugs are given to other people;
5. Look at what the body does "normally"- then either increase or decrease that response;
6. Most of the tricyclic/tetracyclic antidepressants, as well as many of the selective serotonin reuptake inhibitors, serotonin/norepinephrine reuptake inhibitors, and even the mood stabilizers can have some of the chemical "chassis" of those various drugs traced back to the dyes that "change cells"- notably, summer blue, methylene blue, and those dyes are related to the phenothiazine antipsychotic medications like Thorazine (see chapter X); and,
7. The barbiturate medications, like phenobarbital, were used to treat depression.

Just how effective are antidepressants?

Surveys of treatment research indicate the impact of antidepressant medications may be no better than placebo (Mayberg, Silva, Brannan, Tekell, Mahurin, McGinnis, & Jerebek, 2002; Moncrieff, Wessely, & Hardy, 2004). Of note is that the Mayberg report focused on neuroanatomical responses as suggested by the use of various brain scanning techniques. The research proposed to have found increased "activity" in the cortex accompanied by decreases in limbic regions in patients who responded to either Prozac or to a placebo, and postulated that this pattern of changes may be necessary for therapeutic response. Refer to the discussion in page 4 regarding the controversies of neuroimaging (Uttal.)

However, patients in the Mayberg report who responded to fluoxetine also experienced unique changes in lower areas - brainstem, striatum and hippocampus - thought to confer additional advantage in sustaining the response long-term and preventing relapse. Keeping to the research, Mayberg et al reported: "Our findings do not support the notion that antidepressants work merely via a placebo effect. Patients on active medication who failed to improve did not sustain the brainstem, striatal and hippocampus changes unique to antidepressant responders."

Quickly, here are the study design and outcomes:

In the randomized, double blind trial, 17 middle-aged men, hospitalized for unipolar depression, received either Prozac or placebo for 6 weeks. Rating scales revealed that 4 of the men responded to placebo and another 4 showed comparable improvement with the active medication. Nine patients failed to get better.

And the results of the studies?

"Treatment with placebo is not absence of treatment, just absence of active medication," note the researchers, citing possible therapeutic benefits of a change in environment and the supportive, therapeutic milieu of an inpatient psychiatric ward."

One has to wonder if Dr. Uttal might also suggest that the PET scans had a therapeutic effect!

More from the NIMH regarding PET scans, depression, and treatments:

PET scans traced the destination of a radioactive form of glucose - the brain's fuel - to detect brain activity patterns. After 6 weeks, brains of men who responded to either treatment showed "remarkable concordance." Activity increased in prefrontal cortex, posterior cingulate, premotor, parietal cortex, and posterior insula, but activity decreased in subgenual cingulate, parahippocampus, thalamus and hypothalamus.

And what else?

Men who responded to Prozac, in addition, showed changes in certain lower brain areas -- brainstem, hippocampus, striatum and anterior insula. Brain areas activated in the fluoxetine responders were also somewhat larger.

The brain stem and hippocampus appear to have important input in sustaining the cortical/limbic changes, suggest the researchers, who note that absence of changes in these lower brain areas in placebo responders may render those placebo responders to be at higher risk for relapse, which several previous clinical studies had suggested.

And now the comparison between medications!

Although both placebo and antidepressant responders showed increased activity in the posterior cingulate at 6 weeks, this change had already occurred in placebo responders at 1 week. Together with other evidence, this suggests that the ability to increase activity in the posterior cingulate may be an early indicator of a brain's capacity to change and respond to treatment, says Mayberg. Finally, from Dr. Mayberg's research, medications that take a "bottom up" approach or non-drug, cognitive "top-down" interventions should work equally well. However, a need for progressively more aggressive treatments could signal "poor adaptive capacity" in the cortex/limbic network found to change in responders (Mayberg.)

Note that this short discussion regarding the effectiveness of antidepressants is not meant to sound as if these medications do not "work" for some people. Obviously, some patients do get benefit from the employment of these medications for depression. There are researchers who might disagree with the reports listed above, suggesting that both SSRIs and TCAs are effective choices for therapeutic use in patient with depression (von Wolff, Hölzel, Westphal, Härter, & Kriston, 2013; Anderson, 2000; Peveler, Kendrick, Buxton, Longworth, Baldwin, Moore, Chatwin, Goddard, Thornett, Smith, Campbell, & Thompson, 2004).

Different classes of antidepressants include monoamine oxidase inhibitors (MAOIs), tricyclic antidepressants (TCAs), tetracyclic antidepressants, selective serotonin reuptake inhibitors (SSRIs),serotonin/norepinephrine reuptake inhibitors (SNRIs), and atypical antidepressants.

Monoamine oxidase inhibitors

Monoamine oxidase inhibitors (MAOIs) are antidepressants that have been around for a long time. Some examples of MAOIs include phenelzine (Nardil), tranylcypromine (Parnate), isocarboxazid (Marplan), and selegiline (EmSam, Eldepryl) - the former, a transdermal patch, is FDA approved to treat depression; the latter is used to treat Parkinson's Disease.

How do MAOIs work? MAOIs are thought elevate the levels of neurochemicals in the brain synapses by inhibiting monoamine oxid**ase**, the main enzyme that breaks down neurochemicals such as norepinephrine. Keep the enzyme from chewing up norepinephrine- the "tiger chemical" involved in the "fight" of the fight or flight response, and there would be more tiger chemical. And when one is being chased by a tiger, one is not depressed! Get it?

MAOIs also impair the ability to break down tyramine, (another monoamine- understand that monoamine oxidase inhibitors can affect quite a few monoamines, not only those involved in psychopharmacology. Tyramine is a monoamine found in aged cheese, wines, most nuts, chocolate, and other foods. Ingestion of tyramine-containing foods by a patient taking an MAOI drug can cause elevated blood levels of tyramine and dangerously high blood pressure. Of note is that this amino acid, tyramine, cannot cross the blood-brain barrier, so any clinical presentations of the interaction would be nonpsychoactive peripheral sympathomimetic effects, like an increase in blood pressure or even the commencement of a headache.

If a patient takes a MOAI, there may be a clinical presentation best described as an "amphetamine-like" stimulatory effect. Remember how MOAIs are thought to "work"- the antidepressant effect is presumed to be caused by the irreversible and potent suppression of MAO, which in turn raises the concentration of brain monoamines (norepinephrine, epinephrine, serotonin, and dopamine.)

Ah! And now the reader is starting to understand these neurotransmitters! Stimulants by definition "stimulate the release of dopamine!" That is the reason that stimulant medications are called "stimulants!"

So...

If a patient takes a stimulant, that patient's dopamine levels rises in the synaptic cleft. If the normal enzymatic degradation of dopamine in the synaptic cleft is reduced by using MAOIs, the dopamine levels rise! Either way, dopamine levels rise.[54]

Drug interactions with MAOIs can also be a problem. MAOIs also can interact with over-the-counter cold and cough medications like pseudoephedrine (Sudafed) to cause dangerously high blood pressures.

---

[54] These are two separate and distinct mechanisms of action, but both result in the same increase in dopamine availability, dopamine activity, dopamine, whatever!

74

Because of these potentially serious drug and food interactions MAOIs are usually only prescribed after other options have failed. Often heard on television commercials for prescription medications is the phrase: "Don't take this drug if you are taking MAO inhibitors..."

Continuing with the ongoing theme of this book, not all MAOIs will be discussed in detail, due to the similarities in the mechanism of action. Indeed, there may be some differences in half-life, absorption, duration of action, but this book is focusing on the "way these drugs work."

Phenelzine (Nardil)
Classification: MAO inhibitor, hydrazine MAOI.

Used as: Antidepressant

This medication had been stated to be effective in treating the depressed patient clinically characterized as "atypical" or as having "nonindigenous" or "neurotic" depression.

Drug comparisons:

Phenelzine is a little cheaper than tranylcypromine (Parnate) - another MAOI. Phenelzine is seldom a first-choice medication for depression; may have a better benefit for headache relief than other antidepressants. Remember, one must be very careful taking phenelzine (Nardil) with the foods that contain tyramine due to the higher risk of food interactions (Camembert or Bleu Cheese, Chianti wine, and others) as well as a greater severity of untoward side effects.

Remember, too, that inhibition of MAO increases concentrations of several "monoamines," like serotonin, dopamine (within presynaptic neurons and at receptor sites), norepinephrine, and epinephrine. Phenelzine may prolong the effects and activity of many medications by inhibiting microsomal drug-metabolizing enzymes.

Of interest is that this drug does require a significant "wash out" period before institution of any drug that might interact due to continued MAO inhibition (about 2 to 3 weeks). The duration of action of phenelzine is 2 weeks; the onset of action is about 5 to 10 days, and this drug has a half-life is between 1.5 and 4 hours.

Transdermal selegiline (EmSam, Eldepryl)
This MAOI is thought to work on two different MOA receptors:
- It is an inhibitor of MAO_B
- It is a weak inhibitor of MAO_A

Transdermal selegiline (EmSam) was approved by the FDA for depression March 1, 2006.

And, once again, see how much sense these neurotransmitters are beginning to make sense!

Selegiline is already available in tablet and capsule dosage forms for oral use, and the drug is called: "Eldepryl", used to treat Parkinson's disease! Remember, in Parkinson's disease, there are DECREASED levels of- Dopamine!

If the mechanism of action is to "interfere" with the normal enzymatic degradation of dopamine, dopamine levels rise!

Tricyclic antidepressants and tetracyclic antidepressants

Tricyclic antidepressants (TCAs) were developed in the 1950s and 1960s to treat depression. They are called tricyclic antidepressants because their chemical structures consist of three chemical rings.

Hereis the structure of a typical TCA (amitriptyline, Elavil): One can see why this class of drugs are called "tricyclic."

These drugs all have the same information in their Professional Package Insert: "Mechanism of action is not fully understood." However, the proposed mechanism of action is thought to be that TCAs work mainly by increasing the level of norepinephrine in the brain synapses, although TCAs also may affect serotonin levels. Prescribers often use TCAs to treat moderate to severe depression.

How safe are TCAs? TCAs are safe and generally well tolerated when properly prescribed and administered; however, if taken in over-dose, TCAs can cause life threatening heart rhythm disturbances- remember that when faced with a saber-toothed tiger one would see an increase in heart rate!

What about side effects of TCAs? Some TCAs can also have anticholinergic side effects. Anticholinergic side effects are due to blocking of the activity of the nerves responsible for heart rate control, gut motion control, and rate of saliva production.

Chemical structure of amitriptyline (Elavil)

Remember, agonists "increase" and antagonists "decrease" normal bodily functions. So, if the nerves responsible for heart rate control are "blocked" then there can be heart dysrhythmias. If the nerves controlling gut motion are blocked, constipation may occur. And if the nerves that control the rate of saliva production are blocked, the side effect of a dry mouth may occur.

TCAs can produce a feeling of dizziness upon arising, a condition that results from low blood pressure upon standing (orthostatic hypotension). This is why the use of TCAs are not frequently noted in elderly patients, as using these medications might place those patients at higher risks of falling (and constipation.)

There are some researchers who suggest that the tricyclic antidepressants should be considered first line agents in many instances (Coplan, Andrews, Rosenblum, Owens, Friedman, Gorman, & Nemeroff, 1996).

Gregory Simon et al of the University of Washington published a study in the December 2002 *American Journal of Psychiatry* that also suggests that TCAs are better choices, if medication is clinically indicated, for the pregnant client and her fœtus (Simon, Cunningham, & Davis, 2002). Recent studies have suggested that the use of antidepressants (of all classes) during pregnancy might place the fœtus at a higher risk of having a diagnosis of autism (Croen, Grether, Yoshida, Odouli, & Hendrick, 2011), although there are others who disagree about causality. (Rai, Lee, Dalman, Lewis, & Magnusson, 2013)

TCAs should also be avoided in patients with seizure disorders and history of strokes.

Some examples of common tricyclic antidepressants are amitriptyline (Elavil), amoxapine (Asendin), clomipramine (Anafranil), protriptyline (Vivactil), imipramine (Tofranil), desipramine (Norpramin), nortriptyline (Pamelor), doxepin (Sinequan, Silenor) and trimipramine (Surmontil).

Elavil is no longer available in the U.S. (only the generic is available). Second, clomipramine has been re-launched in 2005 under a new Brand name product. Clomipramine is now available as Clomi-calm, and is officially approved by the FDA to treat: Separation anxiety....IN DOGS! OH, yes, there is a Prozac available for dogs, too! This product has a Trade Name of Reconcile, and the treatment is to be accompanied by the BOND™ behavioral training program.

Tetracyclic antidepressants are very similar in action, use, drug interactions, and side effects to tricyclic antidepressants but the tetracyclic antidepressant structures have four chemical rings instead of three. Here is the chemical structure for mirtazapine (Remeron), which will be discussed in a moment:

Examples of tetracyclics include maprotiline (Ludiomil) and mirtazapine (Remeron).

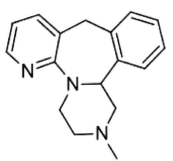

Chemical structure of mirtazapine (Remeron)

More on drug interactions with TCAs- because these medications are significantly protein bound (from imipramine, which can be bound between 63 and 96% to amitriptyline, which is bound between 90 and 97% to protein) there may be significant interactions with other highly protein bound medications. These "other drugs" would include everything from cimetidine (Tagamet) to birth control pills to methylphenidate (Ritalin) to carbamazepine (Tegretol.) There is an interaction- increased blood pressure- with clonidine (Catapres, Kapvay), certain "over the counter" treatments for the common cold, and some medications for breathing difficulties such as albuterol (Ventolin) and epinephrine (adrenaline.)

Can a patient take MOAIs and tricyclic/tetracyclic antidepressants? Well, yes.

Carefully! For refractory patients, one may use TCAs and MAOIs, but understand that there have been severe reactions and fatalities due to hypertensive crises, hyperpyrexia, convulsions, etc., which are seen more often when a TCA is added to established MAOI monotherapy.

Here is a very important note: there is no "therapeutic drug level" of TCAs in the serum. One cannot correlate the blood level of the tricyclic/tetracyclic antidepressants to therapeutic response![55]

Amitriptyline[56]

Classification: Tricyclic antidepressant

Used as: Antidepressant

Drug comparisons:

This drug, the prototype of the class, has (as do other members of the class) more side effects than the newer agents used to treat depression. Because of the many side effects, this class is not used as often as in the past

Note that amitriptyline carries an FDA pregnancy risk category of "C." This means that there are studies that suggest evidence of fetal harm when using this medication in pregnant animals, but either no controlled studies have been done in pregnant women, or, conversely, studies using this drug in pregnant animals have not been done, and studies of pregnant women using the drug are insufficient to reach a conclusion.

It is also important to understand that all pregnancies have a background risk of around 3% for a major birth defect, even when the mother is not taking a drug of any kind (Benfield & Kelley, 2010).[57]

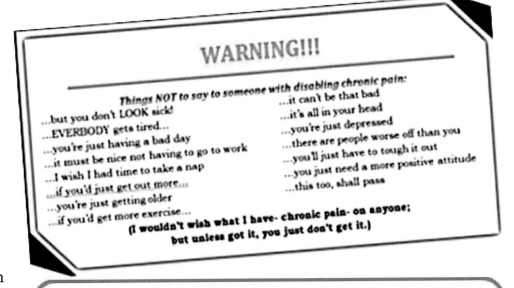

WARNING!!!

Things NOT to say to someone with disabling chronic pain:

...but you don't LOOK sick!
...EVERBODY gets tired...
...you're just having a bad day
...it must be nice not having to go to work
...I wish I had time to take a nap
...if you'd just get out more...
...you're just getting older
...if you'd get more exercise...

...it can't be that bad
...it's all in your head
...you're just depressed
...there are people worse off than you
...you'll just have to tough it out
...you just need a more positive attitude
...this too, shall pass

(I wouldn't wish what I have- chronic pain- on anyone; but unless got it, you just don't get it.)

Modified, and used with the kind permission of Bruce Gerencser.
See his blog at http://www.brucegerencser.net
"The Way Forward"

---

[55] The same statement applies to SSRIs, SRNIs, and other medications. The only psychopharmacological agent where assessing blood levels is even required is lithium, and that is due to the potential toxicity. Having said that, understand that THEROETICALLY as the blood level of medications increases, so does the potential for side effects to appear.

[56] Amitriptyline was marketed as the brand-name product Elavil- only the generic is available in the United States.

Some of these agents, like amitriptyline, may be better suited to the "unapproved" uses of TCAs, such as fibromyalgia, chronic tension headache, diabetic neuropathy, postherpetic neuralgia, and some cancer pain. This class of drugs may require several weeks to show the desired therapeutic response (although the side effects may impart a "bonus" therapeutic effect until the primary therapeutic effect is seen, and may require several titrations to achieve desired therapeutic effect vs. acceptable levels of side effects).

Side effect onset with TCAs? Ah, adverse reactions may appear with the first dose! Consider above that a patient with fibromyalgia who takes a TCA/tetracyclic might benefit from that side effect of drowsiness with the first dose!

Just about done with amitriptyline- all in all, TCAs are safer to use (than barbiturates and benzodiazepines), overdose is easily managed, these are rarely abused, and withdrawal is not a problem. TCAs like amitriptyline and the tetracyclics like mirtazapine are relatively less likely to induce tolerance and dependence.

The onset of action of amitriptyline is usually within an hour, with the peak seen in 2 to 4 hours. There is a significant half-life with this class of drugs, and metabolites are often active- as example, amitriptyline has a half-life of between 10 and 50 hours, but the active metabolite nortriptyline has a 20-100 hour half-life.

These drugs are usually metabolized in the liver, so any medical condition that involves the functioning of the liver, or any other medication that may affect the metabolization capabilities of the liver, might be a concern.

Here is a comparison of chemical structures of common TCAs:

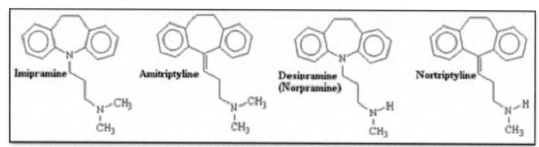

Chemical structures of some common tricyclic antidepressants. Note the "shared" components of the chemical structures.

Mirtazapine (Remeron)
Just a few more words on the tetracyclics-

---

[57] For the rest of this book, the specific Pregnancy Risk Categories of medications will not be addressed unless there is a specific warning. The reader of this book is reminded that:
- The best medication during pregnancy is most likely no medication;
- Risk vs. benefit must be part of the equation- not only for the foetus but also for the mother; and
- Reflect how many women have taking medications while pregnant, but before knowing that pregnancy has commenced.

Mirtazapine (Remeron) has been classified, in some journals, as a: "Norepinephrine-Serotonin Modulator."

Weight gain has been reported in 17% of the patients taking mirtazapine; 7.5% of the patients taking mirtazapine increased body weight by 7%. This is why it is common to see elderly patients in nursing homes receiving this medication- to offset "wasting disorder." Care should be used when using either the TCAs or the tetracyclic medications in the elderly population, due to an increased risk of falls. Constipation and dry mouth are also side effects that may have a significant impact on elderly patients, too.

Activation of manic or hypomanic states appears to be rare (around 0.2%) with either mirtazapine or maprotiline (Ludiomil.)

Mirtazapine (Remeron) is reported to cause significant orthostatic hypotension, and maprotiline (Ludiomil) is not effective in treating panic disorder.

Selective serotonin reuptake inhibitors

Selective serotonin reuptake inhibitors (SSRIs) are medications that increase the amount of serotonin neurochemical in the brain. Although...it is not really known that this is the way that these drugs give a therapeutic effect!

It is time for a little history on SSRIs-

Serotonin (5-hydroxytryptamine, 5-HT) was isolated from the blood as a serum factor that increased smooth muscle tone by Professor D.W. Woolley, a chemist at the Rockefeller Institute. Dr. Woolley described the comparable actions of LSD and serotonin in the cortex of the cat! This finding so intrigued him that he wrote a prophetic book in 1962 entitled *The Biochemical Bases of Psychosis; or the Serotonin Hypothesis about Mental Disease*, and indeed this is the birthdate of the SSRIs! (Woolley, 1962)

SSRIs have been used successfully for decades in the United States to treat depression, and SSRIs have fewer side effects than the TCAs and MAOIs. SSRIs do not interact with tyramine in food like the MAOIs, and do not have orthostatic hypotension and heart rhythm disturbances like traditional antidepressants, such as the TCAs. Therefore, SSRIs are often the first-line treatment for depression.

Let's look at a candy bar[58]-

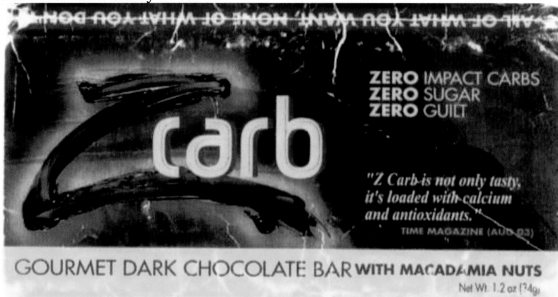

Front of Z-Carb Gourmet Chocolate Bar with Macadamia Nuts

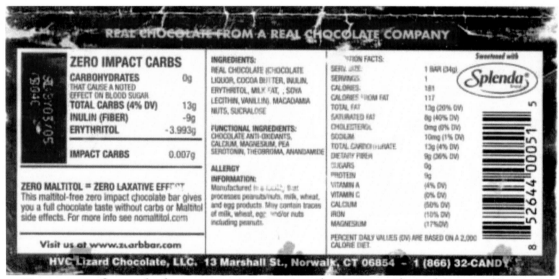

Reverse of candy bar wrapper- Note the "Functional Ingredients"

MAYBE, GENTLE READER, YOU DO UNDERSTAND THESE NEUROTRANSMITTERS BETTER THAN YOU THOUGHT!

See above that this candy bar has a functional ingredient of **serotonin**. Indeed, chocolate is a natural source of serotonin- dark chocolate has an even higher concentration of serotonin than does milk chocolate, and white chocolate? White chocolate is just sweetened cocoa butter, and has no appreciable serotonin concentration.

---

[58] The manufacturer of this product is out of business. The quality of these two scans is poor, and for that, the author apologizes. This is the best image available at the time of the writing of this book

Oh, look above again and see that one of the "functional ingredients" listed is **anandamide**. This is an endogenous cannabinoid neurotransmitter, which means that this chemical theoretically brings about brain activity at the marijuana receptors in the brain.[59]

Some examples of SSRIs include fluoxetine (Prozac and Sarafem[60]), paroxetine (Paxil, Brisdelle, and Pexeva), sertraline (Zoloft), citalopram (Celexa), escitalopram (Lexapro), fluvoxamine (Luvox), and vortioxetine (Brintellix.)

This class of medications is a little different from others previously discussed in this book notably that within the individual drugs one will find few "shared chemical structures" like was seen with the barbiturates, the benzodiazepines, and even the tricyclic/tetracyclic medications. Indeed, this class of drugs stands apart from the other classes, in that these are grouped based solely on the mechanism of action- these all prevent the reuptake of serotonin from the synaptic space into the presynaptic neuron, thereby increasing the amount of available serotonin. Look at the different chemical structures for these medications, but notice that there is little in "shared chassis":

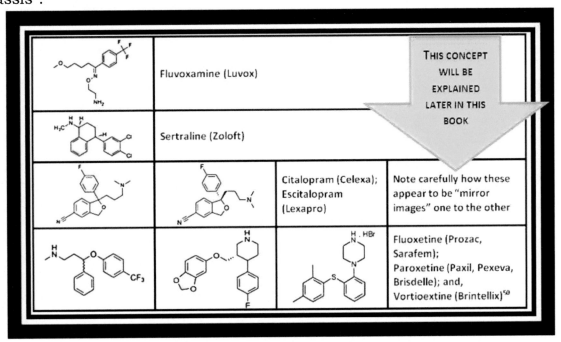

The SSRIs currently available in the United States

Due to the fact that the chemical structures differ from one member of this class of antidepressants to another, theoretically if a patient does not have a therapeutic response from one SSRI, another SSRI could be tried.

---

[59] There is more to this story, too. Anandamide gets its name from the Sanskrit "ananda" which translates to "delight" or "bliss." Psychopharmacology, and the history of psychopharmacology, can be incredibly fascinating!

[60] Sarafem is not approved by the FDA to treat depression, even though it is the same medication as Prozac. Sarafem is approved to treat premenstrual dysphoric disorder, but is being investigated for use in treating PTSD in adults and children, borderline personality disorder, and Raynaud's phenomenon.

How are SSRIs tolerated? These are generally well tolerated and side effects are usually mild. The most common side effects are headache, nausea, and diarrhea.

But these side effects generally dissipate within the first month of use. That is an issue that one should consider in light of other aspects of using these medications. Understand that patients who take these medications may be at a higher risk of suicide within the first few weeks of therapy. In March of 2004 FDA has suggested to prescribers that they monitor their patients for suicidal ideation and attempts within the first few weeks of initiation of therapy.

These issues, specifically:

1. That the side effects happen within the first few weeks of therapy;
2. That the medications may actually take three to four weeks to kick in (have the patient show a clinical response);
3. That the incidence of potential for suicide also may occur in the first few weeks of therapy; and, last,
4. That the side effects appear to wane after about a month...

...may be explained by considering another hypothetical concept discussed early on in this book- homeostasis.

The idea is that the body wants to keep an exquisite balance to maintain optimal functioning so that the body can survive. If the body were to see "too much" norepinephrine (remember the Tiger chemical?) the body would use enzymes (remember all those chemical names having a suffix of "-**ase**"?) to "chew up" the neurotransmitter that the body felt was present in excess.

The same hypothetical concept holds true for all neurotransmitters. If the body feels that there is "too much" (whatever that means) serotonin, the body will use enzymes to decrease the amount of serotonin. Too much dopamine? Enzymes!

So, if the body felt that there was not "enough" serotonin (again, whatever that means) then the body might crave food sources that are rich in either serotonin or chemicals that the body can turn into serotonin. (See the chart found on page 24 showing how the body makes serotonin.)

So what does homeostasis have to do with patients being at a greater risk of suicide within the first few weeks of SSRI therapy?

The patient is depressed and starts taking an SSRI. The levels of serotonin increase, and side effects kick in. The patient may or may not begin to have an improvement in mood. But the body does not like those elevated levels of serotonin, so the body catabolizes- uses enzymes to "eat up" or change the serotonin in an effort to reduce those elevated levels. The levels of serotonin reduce, the side effects go away, but the patient may feel lousy again, and stop taking the SSRI, which (by several different mechanisms, not all of them psychopharmacological) may place the patient at a greater risk of suicide. Remember!

THIS IS <u>ALL</u> HYPOTHETICAL, AND THERE HAVE BEEN NO STUDIES TO ASSERT OR REFUTE THIS THEORY.

Graphically:

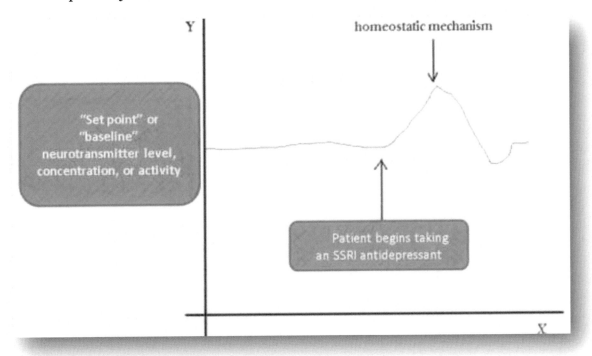

Still more possible side effects with SSRIs:
- ℞ Some patients experience sexual side effects such as decreased libido (with reports up to 70% of the people taking these drugs).
- ℞ Some patients have either a delayed or even an inability to have an orgasm.[61]

Understand that some patients experience tremors with SSRIs, and there is a really serious problem that may occur with SSRIs- Serotonergic Syndrome (also known as "serotonin syndrome") is a serious neurological condition associated with the use of SSRIs. Serotonin syndrome is characterized by high fevers, seizures, and heart rhythm disturbances. Blessedly, serotonin syndrome is rather rare.

Another rare side effect, but one that is seldom discussed with SSRIs, is known as akathisia. This is best described as "feeling jiggly inside." (Sinclair, Christmas, Hood, Potokar, Robertson, Isaac, Srivastava, Nutt, & Davies, 2009)

Here is something interesting- for bipolar patients, the administration of SSRIs may precipitate hypomanic or manic episodes (but one may make the argument that ANY antidepressant, of ANY class, may cause the occurrence of hypomania or mania.) There may be a reason for this, too!
- Remember the similarities in activity between LSD and serotonin in the cat brain?

---

[61] Here is another example wherein one patient's side effect may be another patient's beneficial effect. The drug paroxetine (Paxil, specifically Paxil CR) has been used to treat premature ejaculation in male patients.

Excepting the "old and gold standards" of TCAs, SSRIs as a class are no more expensive than other antidepressants.

Paroxetine (Paxil, Brisdelle, and Pexeva)

Classification: Selective serotonin reuptake inhibitor; phenylpiperidine derivative; racemic bicyclic phthalane derivative.

Brisdelle and Pexeva are paroxetine mesylate- a salt of the same medication as Paxil- paroxetine hydrochloride. Brisdelle and Pexeva are paroxetine mesylate. Refer to the discussion of "salts of drugs" found on page 55 of this book.

Brisdelle is available only in a capsule form, and the dosage is 7.5 mg- a dosage that one does not find available for Paxil or Pexeva.

FDA Approvals[62]	Paxil	Pexeva	Brisdelle
Major Depressive Disorder	X	X	
Obsessive Compulsive Disor	X	?	
Panic Disorder	X	X	
Social Anxiety Disorder	X		
Generalized Anxiety Disorder	X	X	
PTSD	X		
Hot Flashes			X

More on paroxetine, notably the unlabeled uses:
- Bipolar disorder (in conjunction with lithium)
- Chronic headache
- Premature ejaculation
- Fibromyalgia
- Diabetic neuropathy

Still more on paroxetine-

The effect of this drug is thought to be inhibition of the reuptake at the presynaptic clefts of serotonin without affecting other neurotransmitters, resulting in increased serotonin levels.

Pharmacokinetics of paroxetine:
- Time of peak concentration
  - 5-7 hours
- Plasma half-life
  - 24-31 hours

Similarities and differences:

---

[62] As of January 2014.

86

Even though a piperidine derivative, this drug shares few chemical structure similarities with the tricyclic/tetracyclic antidepressants, and may have some effect on acetylcholine receptors.

A significant drug interaction does exist, in that paroxetine should NOT be used with thioridazine (Mellaril), as this medication may reduce the liver's ability to metabolize Mellaril.

Symptoms attributed to Paxil (and other SSRIs) withdrawal have been known as SSRI Discontinuation or Withdrawal Syndrome, and may have an incidence as high at 20% of patients taking these medications. These symptoms might include any, many, several, all, or a few of the following: (Banov, 2010).

- Dizziness
- Vertigo
- Paresthesias
- Visual disturbances
- Lightheadedness
- Diarrhea
- Difficulty walking
- Nausea
- Vomiting
- Fatigue
- Chills
- Muscle pain
- Insomnia
- Shock-like sensations ("jolting electric zaps")
- Worsening depression
- Suicidal thoughts

Paroxetine drug comparisons:

When compared to MAOIs and TCAs, paroxetine, has fewer anticholinergic side effects (dizziness, drowsiness, constipation, dry mouth, dry eye, etc.) -all those nasty side effects that may occur with tricyclic/tetracyclic antidepressants.) Paroxetine has little sedation, like the antihistamines do, and few cardiotoxic untoward effects (including orthostasis.)

Paroxetine HCl (Paxil) may have an incidence of more CNS side effects, like:

- ❖ Insomnia;
- ❖ Sleepiness; or,
- ❖ Nervousness

Paroxetine is cost comparable to other antidepressants (with again the notable exception of the older TCAs.)

Citalopram (Celexa)
Classification: Selective serotonin reuptake inhibitor (SSRI).
Used as: Antidepressant.
Unlabeled (investigational) uses include:

Panic disorder	OCD in adolescents	Posttraumatic stress disorder
Generalized anxiety disorder	Social phobia	Trichotillomania
Premenstrual dysphoric disorder	Impulse aggression in children	
Treatment of psychotic symptoms and behavioral disturbances in nondepressed demented patients		

Effect:

The effect of this medication is not exactly known, but citalopram does seem to inhibit the uptake of serotonin (5-hydroxytryptamine) from the presynaptic clefts without affecting the reuptake of norepinephrine, dopamine, or other neurotransmitters.

Pharmacokinetics of citalopram:
1) Time of peak concentration
   - 2-4 hours
2) Plasma half-life
   - 33-37 hours

Drug comparisons:

Citalopram is partially metabolized in the liver to inactive metabolites.

Note: this drug does not inhibit cytochrome P450 3A4 *in vitro*, so theoretically as a result, it should not affect or be affected by other drugs metabolized by this pathway. But there are other liver pathways, and other drugs which may affect citalopram or that citalopram may affect:

- ℞ If given with certain antifungal medications, the levels of citalopram may increase in the body;
- ℞ If given with β-blockers (remember the discussion early on in this book that the β-blockers are used for many conditions, including anxiety states?) one may see an increase in the effect of the β-blocker (and as such, one should reduce the initial dose of the β-blocker);
- ℞ Give this with carbamazepine (Tegretol and others- remember that carbamazepine is used not only for seizures but also as a mood stabilizer), and one might see an increase in the levels of citalopram and a decrease in the levels of carbamazepine;
- ℞ Take citalopram with imipramine (Tofranil, the first tricyclic antidepressant) and one might see an increase in one of the metabolites of imipramine (specifically, desipramine, which, incidentally, is the brand name TCA known as Norpramin) by 50%;
- ℞ Use lithium with citalopram? One might see an increase in the serotonin effects of citalopram;
- ℞ Take some antibiotics, like erythromycin, clarithromycin, or other "macrolide" and one might see an increase in in citalopram levels; and,

℞ Give citalopram with an MAOI, well, that is just dangerous!

Stereoisomerism explained, and why this is important to this book and psychopharmacology (and, candidly, pharmacology, too!)

Escitalopram (Lexapro)

If written in pharmacy notation...

The chemical name for Lexapro would be: **S-citalopram.**

The capitalized, italicized "**_S_**" is pharmacy shorthand for "sinister"- Latin for "left"

You've heard of other "_S_" drugs-

Nexium is "esomeprazole" (_S_-omeprazole), and is the "left hand side" of Prilosec.

Even Lunesta is the "sinister" side of the molecule: Eszopiclone. Get it? "_S_-zopiclone!"

An example or two of some "right hand side" drugs?

- ✓ **Dextro**amphetamine (Dexedrine) is the right hand side of amphetamine!
- ✓ **Dex**methylphenidate (Focalin) is the right hand side of methylphenidate (Ritalin)!
- ✓ A drug (not discussed in this book other than right now) used to treat daytime sleepiness and narcolepsy is the medication modafinil (Provigil.) Modafinil is being succeeded by armodafinil (Nuvigil) - the "**ar**-"represents the right hand side of modafinil.
- ✓ One may encounter an artificial sweetener, Splenda. "Tastes like sugar because it is made from sugar." Absolutely! Splenda contains **dex**trose, the right hand side of sucrose!

89

This description of "left hand side" and "right hand side" or even "mirror images" is not **_technically_** correct. However, for the purpose of this book- a **_Primer_**- the reader is asked to allow this metaphorical, not completely accurate, representation. The actual definition of a stereoisomer is that the chemical structures have the same atom-to-atom connections, but nonsuperimposable shapes. Understand that just like people, a computer, this book- anything in nature- objects occupy space, and in three dimensions, not two. But even in two dimensions (height and width) you can appreciate that what appears to be two discrete chemical structures is actually the same chemical. As example, look at water- good old H_2O (two hydrogen atoms attached to one oxygen atom.) You will see two images of water:

Even though both of the above are H_2O (water) they have different configurations in space. But they are still both water! See the images below for some more accurate representations of stereoisomers, but remember, it is only the concept that is considered in this book:

EXAMPLES OF THE FOUR KINDS OF STEREOISOMERS

Why the discussion of stereoisomerism and citalopram and escitalopram? Well, the reason is that the FDA has issued a warning about citalopram (Celexa).

As of March of 2012, FDA says that citalopram should not be used in dosages greater than 40 mg per day for any patient and not above 20 mg per day for elderly patients, due to heart dysrhythmias (U.S. Department of Health & Human Services, U.S. Food and Drug Administration, 2012). This warning further clarified a similar warning that the FDA issued regarding citalopram in August of 2011.

It is the experience of this author (as a pharmacist and as a psychologist) that after this warning was issued, many prescribers began moving patients from citalopram (Celexa) to escitalopram (Lexapro.) Understand that the FDA issues warning for specific individual products- and it is the opinion of this author that a similar warning will be forthcoming for escitalopram (Lexapro), most likely that escitalopram not be used for any patient in a dose greater than 20 mg per day, and for elderly patients not to exceed 10 mg per day. This is NOT FDA policy as of the writing of this book, however. It is notable that Magellan Health services has developed "A Patient's Handout for Citalopram/Escitalopram and the FDA Warning" that pretty much states that the "left hand side" of the drug may have similar issues regarding heart dysthymias as the racemic citalopram (Magellan Health Services, n.d.)

Back to escitalopram (Lexapro)-

Classification: Selective serotonin reuptake inhibitor, and like citalopram a napthylamine derivative

Used as (FDA approvals and investigational): Antidepressant; generalized anxiety disorder; PTSD; panic disorder (see below); and appears to also reduce comorbid anxiety states.

Effect:

Well, pretty much the same as citalopram.

A rather "neat" drug in that it is the s-isomeric form of citalopram, a move that was suggested to increase the efficacy to such a level that "one size fits all" for dosing. Indeed, when this product was launched, the manufacturer said it was such a "clean" drug that the dose was 10 mg for everyone, for every condition. This medication is now available as a 5mg tablet, a 10 mg tablet, a 20 mg tablet, and a liquid.

The editors of the internationally respected *Medical Letter On Drugs and Therapeutics* concluded in their September 30, 2002 review of the drug that:

> "Escitalopram (Lexapro), the active enantiomer of citalopram (Celexa), is effective for treatment of depression, but it has not been shown to be more effective, more rapid-acting or less likely to cause adverse effects, including sexual dysfunction, than citalopram or any other SSRI ("Escitalopram (Lexapro) for depression," 2002).

There are some more cautions, and these apply equally to citalopram and escitalopram:

- Should not be taken with MAOIs, and caution is recommended if given with TCAs

Regarding other FDA approvals, drug maker Forest Laboratories Inc. said that the U.S. Food and Drug Administration has turned down for a second time its bid to sell the antidepressant Lexapro as a treatment for panic disorder.

The company said it is reviewing the FDA's response in order to determine how to proceed regarding the drug, which is now used to help treat depressive and anxiety disorders in adults,

The reason for the FDA denial?

Forest Labs first submitted its application for the panic disorder indication in 2003.

The FDA said it was not approvable due to concerns about whether trial methods and analysis proved that the drug was effective (Hoffman, 2005).

Major side effects of escitalopram include, well, pretty much what one might expect from citalopram:

℞ Nausea	℞ Ejaculatory problems
℞ Drowsiness	℞ Fatigue
℞ Insomnia	℞ Increased sweating

Drug comparisons:

There is little sedation, and little cardiotoxicity, and one does not often hear reports of this medication causing orthostatic hypotension.

Fluoxetine (Prozac, Sarafem)

Classification: Selective serotonin reuptake inhibitor; antidepressant.

Used as (here are the official FDA approvals):

- To treat major depressive disorder in adults and children 8-18 years of age;
- Obsessive-compulsive disorders in adults and children 8-18 years of age;
- Long-term treatment of binge-eating and vomiting behaviors in moderate to severe bulimia nervosa;
- Short-term treatment of panic disorder in adults with or without agoraphobia;
- Combined with olanzapine (Zyprexa)[63] for acute treatment of depressive episodes associated with bipolar I disorder in adults[64];
- Combined with olanzapine (Zyprexa)[62] for short-term treatment of treatment-resistant depression in adults who do not respond to 2 separate trials of different antidepressants of adequate dose and duration[63]; and,
- Premenstrual dysphoric disorder (Sarafem, specifically.)

And now another "special" use:

Fluoxetine as the product Zydis ODT has Orphan drug status to treat autism (Merriman, 2012).

More on fluoxetine, now the unlabeled (off-label, or investigational) uses:

☒ Alcoholism	☒ Levodopa-induced dyskinesia
☒ Anorexia nervosa	☒ Fibromyalgia
☒ Borderline Personality Disorder	☒ Raynaud's phenomenon
☒ Cataplexy	☒ Diabetic neuropathy
☒ Chronic daily headache, tension type	☒ GAD
☒ Migraine prophylaxis	

Effect:

Well, the therapeutic effect is not exactly known, but fluoxetine does seem to inhibit the uptake of serotonin (5-hydroxytryptamine) from the presynaptic clefts without affecting the reuptake of norepinephrine or other neurotransmitters, just like most of the other SSRIs.

Pharmacokinetics of fluoxetine:

1) Time of peak concentration
   - 6-8 hours
2) Plasma half-life
   - 2-3 days; the metabolite (norfluoxetine) 7-9 days

---

[63] Eli Lilly has a drug that combines fluoxetine (Prozac) and olanzapine (Zyprexa). This product is known as Symbyax.

[64] Note well that fluoxetine (Prozac) as a monotherapy is NOT approved to treat depressive episodes of bipolar I disorder in adults, nor is fluoxetine (Prozac) approved as monotherapy for treatment-resistant depression.

- With chronic dosing, the half-life may be anywhere between 4 to 16 days to clear the norfluoxetine
  - ⚖ That long half-life of the active metabolite, norfluoxetine, may have therapeutic benefits.
  - ⚖ As example, if a patient is suicidal and there is a question about whether or not that patient is taking the medication correctly
  - ⚖ Also, cessation of therapy is easier as the body "tapers" off the norfluoxetine over an extended period of time, allowing daily evaluations of mood

Drug comparisons:

Some patients may have concerns, as this drug has gotten some "bad press" which may or may not interfere with the patient's therapeutic response, notably suicide reports.

Fluoxetine does, for some patients, appear to be as effective in treating depression as the TCAs, maprotiline, or trazodone.

Side effects of fluoxetine:

Fluoxetine seems to causes less sedation than other antidepressants. As a matter of fact, some patients have difficulty sleeping after using fluoxetine (or any of the SSRIs.) That is why indeed, sometimes trazodone is added to the pharmacotherapy if the client is having trouble sleeping.

Cardiotoxicity is not a problem like with the TCAs.

Fluvoxamine (Luvox)

Classification: Selective serotonin reuptake inhibitor; this is an aralkylketone derivative (does not have similar chemical structure to other SSRIs).

Used as a treatment for:

Obsessive compulsive disorder   Social anxiety disorder

Interesting that the tablets (not capsules) are FDA approved to treat OCD in adults, adolescents, and children, but that the approval is based on DSM-III criteria, not DSM-IV, DSM-IV TR, or the new DSM-5.

Fluvoxamine is also used for the unlabeled, and hence, like all unlabeled uses, investigational treatment of:

Depression;	
Panic disorder;	Social phobia;
Generalized Anxiety Disorder (GAD);	PTSD;
Premenstrual Dysphoric Disorder (PMDD);	Bulimia nervosa;
Nocturnal enuresis (rather like using imipramine- Tofranil- to treat bed-wetting)	
Autism (most often for the compulsivity component of autism, the "Restricted Repetitive Behaviors" listed in the DSM-5) (DSM-5)	

94

Effect:

Pretty much like all the other SSRIs, in that the mechanism of action is not exactly known, but does seem to inhibit the uptake of serotonin (5-hydroxytryptamine) from the presynaptic clefts without affecting the reuptake of norepinephrine or other neurotransmitters. This medication does appear to be more potent in the serotonin reuptake than sister products- but recall that this "increase in serotonin reuptake" has not been correlated with increased efficacy in treating depression.

Pharmacokinetics:

1) Time of peak concentration
   - 2 to 8 hours
2) Plasma half-life
   - 15 to 26 hours

There are few or no anticholinergic or antihistaminic side effects, and fluvoxamine is not likely to cause orthostatic hypotension.

Sertraline (Zoloft)

Classification: a selective serotonin reuptake inhibitor; a napthylamine derivative.

FDA approved uses include:

Major depressive disorder as defined in the DSM-III	**Obsessive-compulsive disorders in adults and children, as defined in the DSM-III-R**
Posttraumatic stress disorder in men and women as defined in the DSM-III-R (getting rather silly with all the different versions of the DSM, is it not?)	**Premenstrual dysphoric disorder, this time as defined in both the DSM-III-R and the DSM-IV**
Social anxiety disorder (social phobia) as defined by the DSM-IV	**Panic disorder, with or without agoraphobia, this time as defined in the DSM-IV**

Sertraline (Zoloft) investigational or unapproved uses include:

- ℞ Nocturnal enuresis (bed-wetting)
- ℞ Hot flashes in men and women (yes, men can experience these, too; if the male patient has an estrogen-dependent tumor and is taking an anti-estrogen, that male patient will experience hot flashes)
- ℞ Cholestatic pruritus (a skin rash that can occur with, oh, most liver diseases)

Effect:

This drug is thought to inhibit the reuptake at the presynaptic clefts of serotonin without affecting other neurotransmitters, resulting in increased serotonin levels.

Pharmacokinetics of sertraline (Zoloft):

1) Time of peak concentration

- 6-8 hours
2) Plasma half-life
- 27 hours

Drug comparisons:

Generally well tolerated, as are members of this entire class. Once again, due to the fact that the chemical structure of sertraline is different from other members of this class of antidepressants, it can be tried in patients who do not have a therapeutic response from other SSRIs.

Perhaps this may not be not a good endorsement...

Notable in that this is the drug that Mike Tyson stated publicly: "I'm on Zoloft to keep me from killing y'all." (ABC News, 2000)

Drug comparisons:

Differs structurally from the classic TCAs, and compared with TCAs and MAOIs, sertraline has little incidence of anticholinergic side effects, little sedation, little cardiotoxicity, and few reports from patients about orthostatic hypotension

Still more comparisons:

Sertraline, like fluvoxamine, may have a likelihood of causing adverse nervous system effects, such as:

- Nervousness
- Somnolence
- Insomnia

- Activation of hypomania or a full blown mania in the bipolar client

Suicide risk with SSRIs (and other antidepressants)

There was some bad press regarding paroxetine and other antidepressants, within different "classes," when used in adolescents. The Food and Drug Administration (FDA) on June 19, 2003 stated it was reviewing reports of a possible increased risk of suicidal thinking and suicide attempts in children and adolescents under the age of 18 treated with the drug Paxil for major depressive disorder (MDD). (Carrey & Virani, 2003) Although the FDA had not completed its evaluation of the new safety data, FDA recommended that Paxil not be used in children and adolescents for the treatment of MDD. There is currently no evidence that Paxil is effective in children or adolescents with MDD, and Paxil is not currently approved for use in children and adolescents. FDA advises that the caretakers of pediatric patients- and those pediatric patients are already receiving treatment with Paxil for MDD talk to their doctor before stopping use of the drug.

Note well that, once again, because a drug is "approved" for use in the U.S., prescribing practitioners may prescribe those drugs for unapproved uses on even unapproved and untested patients!

However, look at the "truth" about the FDA suicide report:

- Over 4,400 children participated in trials
- None of the children committed suicide

There was a small, but statistically significant increase in suicidal ideation and attempts in the paroxetine treated group (3% vs. 1% for controls), and 109 cases were said to be "related." (Whatever THAT means!) Suicidal thoughts in Paxil's reports were classified as being "emotional lability."

Adding to the suicide controversy-

A research study in the May 25, 2005 Journal of the American Medical Association (Kessler, Berglund, Borges, Nock, & Wang, 2005) demonstrated that the huge increase in SSRI therapy during the 1990's produced no diminution in suicidal thoughts, plans, gestures, or attempts; however, and, interestingly enough, the FDA now recommends ALL SSRIs approved to be used to treat depression carry this warning.

THE FDA REVIEW IS DONE!

BETHESDA, MD.   Sept 14, 2004 (USA Today, Health and Behavior. The Associated Press, 2004).

> *The use of some antidepressant drugs appears linked to an increase in suicidal behavior in some children and teenagers, a U.S. advisory panel concluded. The committee said evidence from two dozen clinical trials of nine of the newest antidepressants showed children treated with the drugs were more likely to report suicidal thoughts or actions. Again, no suicides occurred during the trials. The panel of outside medical experts was debating if the risk applied to all of the*

newest antidepressants under review, and which, if any, need stronger warnings. Most of the drugs in question are selective serotonin reuptake inhibitors, or SSRIs.

Concluding from that review:

A U.S. Food and Drug Administration analysis concluded two or three out of every 100 young people treated with antidepressants might be at higher risk of suicidal behavior.

Millions of children are treated with various antidepressants, although only Eli Lilly and Co.'s Prozac is approved for treating pediatric depression,

Which drugs were reviewed by the FDA?

The drugs under review include GlaxoSmithKline PLC's Paxil and Wellbutrin, Eli Lilly's Prozac, Bristol-Myers Squibb's Serzone, Pfizer Inc.'s Zoloft, Forest Laboratories Inc.'s Celexa and Lexapro, Wyeth's Effexor, Solvay's Luvox and Akzo Nobel's Remeron.

And as a result of that review, all antidepressants must carry a "black box" warning, the government's strongest safety alert, linking the drugs to increased suicidal thoughts and behavior among children and teens taking them, the Food and Drug Administration [advisory panel] said:

Because the warnings are seen primarily by doctors, the agency also is creating a medication guide for patients to advise them of the risk.

Dr. Lester Crawford, acting FDA commissioner at the time, said the agency sought to balance the increased risk of suicidal thoughts and behavior against the known benefits of treating depression in children. (U.S. Food and Drug Administration: News and Events. FDA News Release, 2004)

The FDA Commissioner's statement, concluded:

"We continue to believe, however, that these drugs provide significant benefits for pediatric patients when used appropriately." Dr. Crawford said the new labeling warns of the "risk of suicidality and encourages prescribers to balance this risk with clinical need"

The pharmacy manufacturers disagreed, however.

On the same day as this FDA announcement, Eli Lilly issued a prepared statement regarding Prozac in response, warning that the black box label may "...cause doctors not to prescribe it for patients who need it and stop some patients from seeking treatment for their children." The warning label may have a "dangerous effect," the statement from Lilly read (U.S. Today, 2014).

"(Prozac's) safety and efficacy is well-studied, well documented and well-established. Prozac is among the most-studied medications in history."

Note that in those 24 trials involving the 4,400 patients, researchers found that Celexa, Prozac, and Zoloft posed "lower risks" for children, while Luvox, Effexor, and Paxil had higher risks[65].

The outcome of all this is that these warnings will be carried by all antidepressants.

---

[65] That number, 4,400 sounds like a significant number, does it not? But remember, those 4,400 patients were represented by 24 studies, and 9 drugs. Do the math: 4,400÷24÷9= 20.3 persons theoretically could have taken the individual drugs (assuming that there was parity among the drugs and studies.)

Serotonin Norepinephrine Reuptake Inhibitors

Drugs from this class include:
1. Duloxetine (Cymbalta)
2. Venlafaxine (Effexor)[66]
3. Desvenlafaxine (Pristiq)
4. Milnacipran (Savella)
5. Levomilnacipran (Fetzima)

What is different about these from others we've already seen?

The major differences between these SNRIs are their individual specificity for receptors and the significances of the side effect profiles. Remember with the serotonin/norepinephrine reuptake inhibitors, the goal of these therapies has been to provide "dual action" coverage to effect reuptake inhibition of both serotonin and norepinephrine.

A comparison of the SNRIs:

Duloxetine (Cymbalta)

Classification: SNRI; antidepressant.

This product was approved by the FDA on August 4, 2004. This medication was approved by the FDA to treat diabetic peripheral neuropathy (09/07/2004). It is important to note that Cymbalta was the first drug EVER "officially approved" for this condition by the FDA.[67]

Cymbalta was officially approved for maintenance treatment of Major Depressive Disorder in November of 2007, for management of fibromyalgia in July of 2008, , to treat Generalized Anxiety Disorder in November of 2009, and on November 5, 2010 to treat Chronic Musculoskeletal Pain.

There is an "unapproved use" for duloxetine in the United States (well, actually, this is used for several "unapproved" conditions, but this one is interesting): treatment for stress urinary incontinence. Approval for Yentreve (same drug- duloxetine) was given August 15, 2004 in the European Union.

Compare this use and remember that the theoretical mechanism of action is to increase the availability of both norepinephrine and serotonin in the synaptic space. Sounds a little like imipramine (Tofranil), does it not? The reader will recall that Tofranil is used "off-label" in the United States to treat bedwetting. See the similarities? There could be a similar argument for comparison of Cymbalta for the various pain and depressive disorders listed

---

[66] Effexor is only available in the US as the Extended Release form; the generic is still available in the immediate-release tablet.)

[67] Some readers of this book may state: "Hey, wait a minute! Patients have been using gabapentin (Neurontin) to treat diabetic peripheral neuropathic pain for years!" Gabapentin was approved by the FDA to treat neuropathic pain, while duloxetine (Cymbalta) was the first drug approved to treat **diabetic** peripheral neuropathic pain.

above- is it not true that Elavil is also used for these conditions, and also is thought to "work" on norepinephrine (the Tiger Chemical) and maybe serotonin, just as Cymbalta is thought to work on both norepinephrine and serotonin?

Drug comparisons:

There are fewer reports of side effects (weight gain, abnormal ejaculation, or impotence) than with comparator SNRIs; this drug seems to have a better specificity for neurotransmitters than clomipramine or imipramine, and has been reported to have fewer incidences of side effects than fluoxetine, paroxetine, clomipramine, and imipramine. This drug does lack the orthostatic side effect seen in the TCAs/tetracyclics.

This is what a "black box" warning looks like! (Edited for content by the author of this book.)

> *Suicidality in Children and Adolescents — Antidepressants increased the risk of suicidal thinking and behavior (suicidality) in short-term studies in children and adolescents with major depressive disorder (MDD) and other psychiatric disorders.*
>
> *Anyone considering the use of Cymbalta or any other antidepressant in a child or adolescent must balance this risk with the clinical need.*
>
> *Patients who are started on therapy should be observed closely for clinical worsening, suicidality, or unusual changes in behavior.*
>
> *Families and caregivers should be advised of the need for close observation and communication with the prescriber.*
>
> *Cymbalta is not approved for use in pediatric patients. (See WARNINGS and PRECAUTIONS, Pediatric Use.)*
>
> *Pooled analyses of short-term (4 to 16 weeks) placebo-controlled trials of 9 antidepressant drugs (SSRIs and others) in children and adolescents with major depressive disorder (MDD), obsessive compulsive disorder (OCD), or other psychiatric disorders (a total of 24 trials involving over 4400 patients) have revealed a greater risk of adverse events representing suicidal thinking or behavior (suicidality) during the first few months of treatment in those receiving antidepressants.*
>
> *The average risk of such events in patients receiving antidepressants was 4%, twice the placebo risk of 2%. No suicides occurred in these trials.*

Venlafaxine (Effexor)

Classification: Selective serotonin reuptake inhibitor; selective noradrenaline reuptake inhibitor; a very weak inhibitor of dopamine reuptake; napthylamine derivative.

Used as: Antidepressant; for treatment of GAD (the extended-release has this approval); treatment of Social Anxiety Disorder (Social Phobia); and for treatment of panic disorder with or without agoraphobia.

Effect: Blocks norepinephrine (NE) and serotonin (SE) reuptake in the neurons of the CNS.

Pharmacokinetics of venlafaxine-

- Time of peak concentration
    - 2 hours
- Plasma half-life
    - 5 hours (note that this half-life is increased in clients with liver or kidney disease)

Stopping the medication should be accomplished by tapering gradually over a 2 week period (to prevent "discontinuation symptoms").

Drug comparisons:

Venlafaxine is an interesting drug; some researchers suggest that venlafaxine has two levels of antidepressant activity. At low levels, it seems to function as an SSRI, while at higher doses, venlafaxine also appears to inhibit reuptake of norepinephrine; this is a controversial subject of discussion amongst the scientists, as the FDA does not recognize this as an issue (Preskorn, 1999). Indeed, one would expect more of a norepinephrine response, such as an increase in heart dysrhythmias, as the dose increases. As a matter of fact, this medication can cause hypertension at the higher levels, which should be monitored. Regardless of whether the immediate-release dose or the sustained-release dose is used, titration is required. Venlafaxine may cause some mild anticholinergic side effects (dry mouth, constipation, dizziness, etc.) and sedation. Venlafaxine has a low risk of seizure as compared to TCAs and tetracyclic antidepressants.

The FDA MedWatch Warning:

June 29, 2004 — Neonates exposed to venlafaxine (Effexor and Effexor XR, made by Wyeth) late in the third trimester may develop complications immediately upon delivery and require prolonged hospitalization, respiratory support, and tube feeding, according to a warning issued by Wyeth Laboratories, the U.S. Food and Drug Administration (FDA) safety information and adverse event reporting program. (Hassner Sharav, 2004)

The warning also applies to other serotonin and norepinephrine reuptake inhibitors (SNRIs) and selective serotonin reuptake inhibitors (SSRIs)

And from the Medicines and Healthcare Regulatory Agency, December 6, 2004:

Venlafaxine (Efexor- yes, that is how this drug is spelled in Europe.)

The CSM has additionally considered the balance of risks and benefits of Efexor because of concerns about cardiotoxicity and toxicity in overdose.

CSM recommends that treatment with Efexor should only be initiated by specialist mental health practitioners, including GPs with special interest, and there should be arrangements in place for continuing supervision of the patient.

Efexor should not be used in patients with heart disease (e.g. cardiac failure, coronary artery disease, ECG abnormalities including pre-existing QT prolongation), patients with electrolyte imbalance or in patients who are hypertensive.
Patients currently doing well on treatment with venlafaxine can continue to the end of their course. (MHRA cautions against cardiotoxicity of venlafaxine, 2004).

Desvenlafaxine succinate (Pristiq)

Desvenlafaxine (Pristiq) is the "right hand side" of venlafaxine (Effexor), just like Lexapro is the "left hand side" of Celexa.

Wyeth submitted a New Drug Application for treatment of Major Depressive Disorder (MDD) on December 22, 2005, and received official FDA approval to treat adult patients with MDD on March 3, 2008.

Wyeth filed a New Drug Application with the FDA in 2006 for treating vasomotor symptoms associated with menopause (that is a fancy medical phrase for "hot flashes" and received an approvable letter in July of 2007. Note that this was an approvable letter, not an approval. The manufacturer withdrew that request in February of 2010.

Milnacipran (Savella)

Technically, a SNRI, but not approved for depression! Well, not in the US, anyway...

Remember that Cymbalta is approved for chronic pain and fibromyalgia?

Savella is approved for fibromyalgia. Milnacipran inhibits the reuptake of serotonin and norepinephrine in an approximately 1:3 ratio, respectively. Having said that, inhibition of both neurotransmitters simultaneously is thought to work "synergistically" to treat both depression and fibromyalgia. Milnacipran exerts no significant actions on histamine-1 (H1), alpha adrenergic-1 (α1), dopamine-1 (D1), dopamine-2 (D2), and acetylcholine (mACh)[68] receptors, as well as on benzodiazepine and opioid binding sites.[69] Truly, this medication sounds like it was made for older adults in chronic pain. But that is not why milnacipran is mentioned in this book, gentle reader.

---

[68] What this means in plain English is that milnacipran does not cause drowsiness, does not cause patients to fall over upon arising, does not give patients the "hand shaky thing" of Parkinson's Disease or give patients the buzz seen with amphetamines and other stimulants, does not affect the colon/cause dry eye/dry mouth/dizziness.

[69] What this means is that this drug may be co-administered to patients taking medications like pain killers (OxyContin, Vicodin, etc.) and/or benzodiazepine medications (Valium, Xanax, etc.)

Look carefully at the chemical structure of milnacipran:

Milnacipran (Savella)

See the "right hand" and the "left hand" sides of the chemical structure? This is an excellent example of the concept discussed earlier in this book known as "stereoisomerism" that yielded such medications as Lexapro (left hand side of Celexa), Dexedrine (right hand side of amphetamine), Pristiq (right hand side of Effexor), Focalin (right hand side of Ritalin), and others.

Well, now, take that left hand side of milnacipran (Savella) and you get levomilnacipran (Fetzima):

Levomilnacipran (Fetzima™)

Levomilnacipran (Fetzima)

Levomilnacipran is approved by the U.S. Food and Drug Administration (FDA) for the treatment of Major Depressive Disorder (MDD) in adults as of July 2013. And there is nothing more to say, other than it is the left hand side of Savella. Pretty cool, eh?

Atypical antidepressant drugs

Atypical antidepressants are so named in this book because there is a lack of a common mode of action among them, although there is no official "class" of medications called "atypical antidepressant drugs." This concept is used in this book as the readers are familiar with the phrase "atypical antipsychotic drugs"- so this concept is borrowed here.

These medications are neither TCAs (like Elavil) nor SSRIs (like Prozac); but like those more familiar agents, these atypical antidepressants increase the level of certain neurochemicals in the brain synapses. Examples (this is a non-inclusive list) include nefazodone, trazodone (Desyrel, Oleptro), vilazodone (Viibryd) and bupropion (Wellbutrin/Zyban).

Nefazodone[70]

Nefazodone, like the sister drugs trazodone (Desyrel, Oleptro) and vilazodone (Viibryd), is a triazolopyridine derivative. Here is a comparison of the chemical structures of these three triazolopyridine medications:

	Nefazodone
	Trazodone (Desyrel , Oleptro)
	Vilazodone (Viibryd)

Note well that there are several chemical "parts" that are shared between these three chemicals.

Interesting, nefazodone is also very closely related in chemical structure to aripiprazole (Abilify) (Poore, 2014a). The reader of this book will recall that on page 13 and footnote, the history of "where these drugs came from" was addressed. Recall also that most of the antidepressants (and most of the mood

---

[70] Nefazodone was still on the United States market as of 2012, but now only the generic is available.

stabilizers and other psychopharmacological agents) came from a treatment for malaria- summer blue, a dye that, in contact with the skin, would turn skin blue.

Note the "-azo-" part of the generic name nefazodone, as well as the "-pyridine-"part.

"-azo-" chemicals can turn the skin red when contact is made, and "-pyridine-" drugs all share a similar chemical structure, which will be presented.

There is a medication, phenazopyridine (as a prescription medication, known as Pyridium and also available Over-The-Counter, known as Azo Standard), that is used to treat urinary tract irritation.

Patients who take this medication find the urine changes to an orange. That is not exactly correct, the dye in phenazopyridine turns the urine red, but because urine is usually a yellow color, the resulting urinary tint is orange. Oh, and phenazopyridine is usually taken as a result of an infection, and patients with urinary tract infections often have a clinical presentation of a lousy mood!

See how all this comes together? A patient has an infection...give a medication that changes something...use that medication for mood issues!

Psychopharmacology is not that hard- people just make it hard!

Nefazodone has been described as a "serotonin modulator"- and the author of this book has no idea what that means! Serotonin, by definition, will modulate depending on the needs of the patient at any given time.[71] This medication is also described having a mechanism of action whereby there is a potent and selective blocking of postsynaptic serotonin (5-hydroxytryptamine; 5HT) $5HT2_A$ receptors, allthewhile moderately inhibiting serotonin and noradrenaline (norepinephrine) reuptake.

More on nefazodone:

There have been reports of life-threatening hepatic failure with this drug. Indeed, there are only TWO countries in the world where this drug is still allowed to be used: the U.S. and Australia!

Many people (possibly including you, dear Reader) think that this drug is off the market, but no, that is not the case. The manufacturer of the brand-name Serzone had "stopped" distribution of Serzone as of 06/14/2004 due to a class action lawsuit brought by the organization Public Citizen regarding that liver problem. The drug was never recalled by the FDA or the manufacturer, and if pharmacists had Serzone on the drugstore shelves, the medication could be dispensed. This medication is only available in the US as the generic form as of the writing of this book (2014.)

The lawsuit has been resolved. If needed, more information on the settlement is available at:

http://www.drug-injury.com/druginjurycom/2005/09/serzone_mdl_cla.html

---

[71] Reflect back on the concept of "homeostasis" described in text on page 84 and presented graphically on page 85.

Drug comparisons:

Nefazodone has been reported to have fewer cardiotoxic effects than the TCAs/tetracyclics, and can be used with SSRIs to block the untoward sexual side effects. This medication is anxiolytic as well as sedating, and may cause more orthostatic hypotension than the SSRIs. Fewer anticholinergic side effects[72] are encountered by patients with this medication than with some of the other antidepressants.

This medication is about the same cost as other drugs (other than amitriptyline), and do know that if taken with food or milk the absorption of this drug, and hence the bioavailability, is profoundly decreased, so the best way to take nefazodone is on an empty stomach.

Trazodone (Oleptro[73])

This also is described as a "serotonin modulator". Candidly, this drug appears to be more often used for the unlabeled (not FDA approved) uses:

- 50 mg of trazodone with tryptophan 500 mg twice daily has been successful in treating aggressive behavior (O'Neil, Page, Adkins, & Eichelman, 1986; Roy, Hoffman, Dudas, & Mendelowitz, 2013);
- To decrease "cravings" for alcohol, and to treat the symptoms of anxiety and depression seen in the alcoholic client;
- As a somnotic to offset SSRI-induced insomnia;
- To treat panic disorder;
- To treat agoraphobia; and,
- As an adjunct therapy for Male Erectile Dysfunction[74]

Effect:

Not well understood, but the current theory about the mechanism of action of trazodone is that this medication is to inhibit serotonin reuptake, and this medication does also appear to antagonize α-adrenergic receptors and postsynaptic 5HT2 receptors- which means that if someone arises quickly, that person may feel lightheaded (and perhaps faint.) Trazodone does not stimulate the CNS; therefore it is more sedating than nefazodone. Likewise, because there is no CNS stimulation, this drug might better for use as a sedative-hypnotic in clients with addiction problems- as clients cannot get a "buzz" from using trazodone.

The author of this book believes that trazodone is a "lousy" antidepressant (better choices available) but not a bad "sleeper." That this drug appears to have minimal cardiovascular effects, and few anticholinergic side effects, patients seem to tolerate therapy better.

---

[72] Remember: Dizziness, drowsiness, dry mouth, dry eye, constipation, urinary retention, weight gain, orthostatic hypotension, and blurred vision are examples of anticholinergic side effects, and these potential side effects are not as significant a problem with nefazodone, trazodone, or vilazodone.

[73] Oleptro is a once-a-day dosage form of Desyrel; Desyrel is no longer available in the United States- the generic form is still on the market.

[74] Trazodone may cause a side effect known as priapism- a functional and sustainable penile erection.

Trazodone is best taken with food (even if taken at bedtime); absorption is increased by 20%. Note that this is a little different from nefazodone (Serzone), which, if taken with food may cause some decrease in the bioavailability.

Vilazodone (Viibryd)

Vilazodone was originally discovered by Merck KGaA. After early clinical development, the drug was licensed to GlaxoSmithKline (GSK). Clinical testing in Phase II trials yielded unsatisfactory data, so in 2003 GSK walked away from the licensing agreement in 2003 and all rights to vilazodone were returned to Merck KGaA. Continued research suggested that some patients with a specific biomarker, called PGx, did respond to this medication. Development rights were then sold to Genaissance Pharmaceuticals.

Genaissance has developed a genetic (DNA) test that will predict whether or not you will respond to this antidepressant!

This is the field known as "pharmacogenomics"- tailor made medications. Ask why a patient would take a medication that is known to have no effect on that patient, due to genetic issues!

Vilazodone did not get approved by the FDA with that genetic test, for some significant reasons:

1. No insurance company wanted to pay the costs of an expensive genetic test, when a patient could just go to a local large chain pharmacy and get generic citalopram (Celexa) for $4.00 for a one month supply; and,
2. If the patient had a genetic cause for a medication to not have effectiveness, one could make an argument that that patient had a pre-existing condition, and theoretically NO mental health services would be covered.[75]

This drug works as an SSRI and as a 5HT1A agonist

Rather like giving the benefits of a Prozac AND a BuSpar at the same time! Yes, this medication should be taken with food.

The company now marketing Viibryd is Forest Pharmaceuticals.

Bupropion (Wellbutrin, Zyban)

Classification: Antidepressant, a monocyclic amino ketone.

This drug is related to diethylpropion, an old diet pill from the 1990's. The generic form of diethylpropion is still available in the United States as of 2014.

Used as: Antidepressant; Smoking cessation agent (Zyban)
Unlabeled uses:

- ADHD (Wellbutrin)
- Neuropathic pain treatment
- To "enhance weight loss"

---

[75] Theoretically, this topic of a pre-existing condition no longer is a concern due to the parameters of the Affordable Care Act of 2010. (Patient Protection and Affordable Care Act, P.L. 111-148. 2010)

Effect:

Seems to mildly inhibit serotonin, norepinephrine, and dopamine reuptake. This statement is controversial, as the manufacturer and the FDA do not include any serotonin activity as the proposed mechanism of action. However, bupropion has been known to cause serotonin syndrome, so therefore there must be an effect on serotonin, too. (Munoz, 2004; Thorpe, Pizon, Lynch, & Boyer, 2010; Gilman, 2010)

Pharmacokinetics of bupropion

- Time of peak concentration: 2 hours (conventional tablet); sustained-release tablets: 3 hours.
- Plasma half-life (for all forms) is 14 hours.

Drug comparisons:

This drug is less sedating than other medications in the antidepressant class. If insomnia is a problem, consider dosing either of the sustained-release forms (Wellbutrin SR or Wellbutrin XL) at bedtime. No kidding, bedtime! The reason is just how long it takes this medication to enter the system. Obviously, as this medication is related to diet pills, it does not cause weight gain.

There is an increased risk of seizure occurrence with this drug, but this is seen usually with the immediate-release form. The risk appears low and has not been proven with the sustained release preparation. Bupropion does not cause orthostatic hypotension, and has fewer anticholinergic and/or antihistaminic side effects than other agents.

Do note that there are special dosage considerations for patients with liver problems. In patients with "severe hepatic cirrhosis" therapy should be started at a lower dosage and should not exceed 75 mg per day for immediate-release Wellbutrin and should not exceed 100 mg per day OR 150 mg every OTHER day for Wellbutrin SR or Zyban. Persons with kidney impairment have not been evaluated for dosage maximums, but it is "suggested" that the dosage be reduced or given less frequently.

Dosing and Drug comparisons

NOTE "NEW" DOSAGE LIMITS:

No single dose should exceed 150 mg of the regular-release tablets or daily dose of 450 mg.

Dosage recommendations for the sustained-release formulations; for Wellbutrin SR, no single dose should exceed 200 mg, and not more than 400 mg per day; for Wellbutrin XL the maximum daily dose is 450 mg, with no single daily dose exceeding 450 mg.

Dosage recommendations for kids- and remember, these are only "recommendations":

Children and adolescents: limited data available. The suggested dose is 250mg to 300 mg per day for the regular release tablets- but remember that dosages of medications are as individual as the patients who take those medications. For children under the age of 5, safe and effective use has not been established.

The manufacturer's literature lists "hostility" as a side effect in 5.6% of the patients who take this medication. The reason?

DOPAMINE!

Stimulants- the first antidepressants

Yes, stimulants were (and are) used as antidepressants. Candidly, stimulants such as methylphenidate (Ritalin) or dextroamphetamine (Dexedrine) are faster acting than the other antidepressants.

They may be used initially for several weeks in addition to an antidepressant to treat certain patients with severe depression.

But let's look at these in their own class, as psychopharmacological agents used to treat ADHD and ADD. REMEMBER! These are dopamine AGONISTS! Too much dopamine (again, whatever THAT means!) can result in tics, psychosis, mania, etc.

A patient who theoretically has "too much dopamine" may appear to be psychotic. So, that patient would receive a dopamine ANTAGONIST- an antipsychotic medication.

Drugs are (at this time) the mainstay of ADD/ADHD therapy, and the most often encountered class of medications used to treat ADD/ADHD are indeed the stimulants. So, now to have a discussion about stimulant medication-

This book will focus on three classifications of medications used for ADHD/ADD treatment.

1. Amphetamines
2. Methylphenidate products
3. "Other"

Amphetamine

Classification: CNS stimulant. This medication exists as a "racemic" mixture- left hand side and right hand side together.

Used as: Anorexiant (to treat exogenous obesity- a fancy way of saying "a diet pill"; Antinarcoleptic; ADHD.

Effect: CNS activity stimulated by the release of norepinephrine, and at high doses, dopamine is also released.

Time of peak concentration: Therapeutic response seen in one to three hours, however the time to peak is 2 to 4 hours

Plasma half-life: 7 to 8 hours for urinary acidification below pH 5.6; for each 1 unit increase in pH one sees a 7 hour increase in plasma half-life. Normal urinary pH is 6.5 to 8.

When using this medication it is important to monitor weight and growth of the patient.

Drug comparisons:

Amphetamine is a potent psychomotor stimulant; the use of this medication (and any of the other stimulants, for that matter) causes a release of the excitatory neurotransmitters dopamine and noradrenaline (norepinephrine) from storage vesicles in the CNS.

Amphetamine may be sniffed, swallowed, snorted or injected. Amphetamine may induce exhilarating feelings of power, strength, energy, self-assertion, focus and enhanced motivation, and the need to sleep or eat is diminished. Amphetamine administration, which again has an effect on "stimulating the release of dopamine into the synaptic space," typically induces a sense of aroused euphoria, which may last several hours. Unlike cocaine, amphetamine is not readily broken down by the body

Remember: releases dopamine, blocks reuptake, and interferes with monoamine oxidase- the enzyme that Professor D.W. Woolley investigated and was discussed early on in this book (see page 81)

Feelings are intensified, and the user may feel he can take on the world.

Effects are similar with methylphenidate (Ritalin and the many other forms of methylphenidate, to be discussed within a few pages.)

Commentary:

- Millions of doses of amphetamine were taken by soldiers on both sides of World War II
- It was not uncommon for there to be "battlefield psychosis" as a result
  - Remember: "too much" dopamine= psychosis
- Adolf Hitler took daily injections of methamphetamine from his doctor
- One would have to wonder how history would have been different if these drugs were not available...

Dextroamphetamine (Dexedrine)

Classification: Stimulant; Sympathetic amine.

Used as: Antinarcoleptic; to treat ADHD. Understand that the use of amphetamines is not recommended in children younger than 3 years of age (Spratto).

More on dextroamphetamine-

Effect: Releases norepinephrine (the "Tiger chemical"), which stimulates CNS activity, and at high doses, releases dopamine (hence, this is a "stimulant" as it "stimulates" the release of dopamine into the synaptic cleft.)

Drug comparisons:

About twice as potent as the racemic mixture, giving a greater CNS effect and less cardiovascular effects. Indeed, just like amphetamine, the psychopharmacological effects are similar to methylphenidate (Ritalin and others). The elimination half-life is longer than for methylphenidate, but dosing and effectiveness are similar.

Mixed salts of amphetamine (Adderall)

Classification: Central nervous system stimulant; this is a combination of the D-stereoisomer plus racemic mixture of amphetamines (remember the discussion of the "left hand side and right hand side of medications?)[76].

Just like amphetamine, the mixed salts of amphetamine are thought to block the reuptake of norepinephrine and dopamine in the brain.

Approved uses of Adderall: ADHD treatment; approved August 2003 for adult ADHD.

Adderall was only the second drug "approved" for this indication, and on August 14, 2004 Adderall XR was given an approval extension to treat adult ADHD; to treat narcolepsy.

Drug comparisons:

This medication seems to have less cardiovascular effects than amphetamine alone; this drug may require multiple dosing during the day.

There is a sustained-release capsule available.

The rationale for using the mixture?

This drug uses the concept of mixing different forms of amphetamine, with the theoretical basis that a mixture of different types of one drug will allow for better therapeutic results with lesser side effects (notably, the cardiac side effects.) This is rather like the idea of mixing 97 octane gasoline with 93 octane gasoline to get a blended 95 octane- your child- or now even an adult (the engine)- runs a little better, but has fewer knocks.

Obviously, there are similarities with the other stimulants. For example, the side-effect profile of Adderall is similar to that of other psychostimulants, with the most common being:

Stomachaches;	Appetite suppression;
Sleep disturbances; and,	Headaches

But interestingly, parent acceptance is high. What this means is that parents feel that this drug does give benefits to the children. As example, parents of children taking Adderall reported that their children experienced fewer occurrences of anxiety, irritability, and staring/daydreaming compared with those taking placebo.

---

[76] Amphetamine exists as the combination of both the left hand side and the right hand side of the molecule. This is known as a "racemic" mixture. You will recall that dextroamphetamine (literally, "D-amphetamine) is only the right hand side. Adderall is a combination of amphetamine (left and right hand side) and dextroamphetamine (only the right hand side.) in essence: Left, right, and right side of the amphetamine molecule= mixed salts of amphetamine (Adderall.)

Drug comparisons:

As one would expect, the mixed salts of amphetamine would result in stimulation of the CNS, resulting in:

Wakefulness	Diminished sense of fatigue	Increased motor activity
Appetite suppression	Alertness	Mood elevation

And the pharmacokinetics of the mixed salts of amphetamine (Adderall):

Time of peak concentration:

1. One to five hours (immediate-release form)
2. 7 hours (controlled-release form)

Plasma half-life

℞ 14 hours (for both formulations)

Here is some dated information about some of the controversies surrounding the use of psychostimulants, specifically Adderall:

Health Canada suspends the market authorization of ADDERALL XR

Health Canada Online February 9, 2005 (Drugs.com, 2005)

OTTAWA –

Health Canada is informing Canadians that it has instructed Shire BioChem Inc., the manufacturer of ADDERALL XR to withdraw the drug from the Canadian market.

Health Canada has suspended the market authorization of the product due to safety information concerning the association of sudden deaths, heart-related deaths, and strokes in children and adults taking usual recommended doses of ADDERALL and ADDERALL XR. The immediate release form of ADDERALL has never been marketed in Canada.

Health Canada is advising patients who are currently being treated with ADDERALL XR to consult their physician immediately about use of the drug and selecting treatment alternatives.

Health Canada's decision comes as a result of a thorough review of safety information provided by the manufacturer, which indicated there were 20 international reports of sudden death in patients taking either ADDERALL (sold in the United States, not in Canada) or ADDERALL XR (sold in Canada)

Was the Adderall being abused or misused?

> *These deaths were not associated with overdose, misuse or abuse.*

Fourteen deaths occurred in children, and six deaths in adults; there were 12 reports of stroke, two of which occurred in children. However, none of the reported deaths or strokes occurred in Canada

A preliminary review of safety data for the other related stimulants authorized for use in the treatment of ADHD in Canada has been conducted, and in that review, the incidence of serious adverse reactions leading to death was higher in ADDERALL and ADDERALL XR combined than in the other drugs of this class. As a result, the Canadian Health Ministry is seeking information on ALL stimulants. Health Canada has asked manufacturers of other related stimulants approved for the treatment of ADHD to provide a thorough review of their worldwide safety data.

Information updates will be provided by Health Canada as they become available.

Patients taking drugs of the same class for the management of ADHD should NOT discontinue their medication, and should consult with their physician if they have any concerns or questions.

ADDERALL XR, a Central Nervous System (CNS) stimulant, was approved in Canada on January 23, 2004 for the management of Attention Deficit Hyperactivity Disorder (ADHD) in children.

Do understand that this authorization removal was temporary, and Health Canada allowed Adderall XR to return 6 months after that withdrawal. (Canadian Adverse Drug Reaction Monitoring Program (CADRMP), Marketed Health Products Directorate, HEALTH CANADA, 2006)

Thursday, January 12, 2006 the United States FDA began specific reviews about the safety of this class of drugs when used in all patients-although there was no specific action in the United States like there was in Canada (United States Food and Drug Administration, 2006).

Methamphetamine HCl (Desoxyn)

Yes! This medication is still available as a prescription drug in the United States as of the writing of this book (2014.)[77]

Classification: Central nervous system stimulant. Incidentally, chemically this is "desoxyephedrine HCl"[78]- and now you know why ephedrine and (especially!) pseudoephedrine are used in the illegal manufacture of crystal methamphetamine.

Mechanism of action: Blocks reuptake of norepinephrine and dopamine in the brain.

Used as: A treatment for ADHD; this author has had two patients using this medication of recent- one was a patient with AIDS (most likely for energy, as his body was completely tapped out and the other was a dentist with narcolepsy. Methamphetamine HCl is also used to treat exogenous obesity.

According to the manufacturer:

---

[77] There is some confusion, even in the pharmacy industry, about whether or not this is still available. The author called the manufacturer of this product- Recordati Rare Diseases- on 6 February, 2014, and affirmed that this is still in production and still available on the United States Market. Two other internet references (RxList: The Internet Drug Index. Desoxyn, 2013; Express Scripts, Gold Standard, An Elsevier Company, 2009) describe this product as being available, but the 2013 Edition of the Delmar Healthcare Drug Handbook (Spratto) does not list this product. This author also called a retail pharmacy (Kroger Pharmacy in Whiteland, Indiana) on 6 February, 2014, and was told that the manufacturer has discontinued this product. Nope! It is still available!

[78] As one might suspect, methamphetamine is the "right hand side" of oxyephedrine.

🜍 "Do not diagnose this condition [ADHD] with finality when these symptoms are only of comparatively recent origin."

Drug comparisons:

This medication is teratogenic (has been associated with birth defects) and is embryocidal (in animals at doses higher than seen in human therapies). Like the other amphetamine medications, the effects similar to methylphenidate (Ritalin and others.) The elimination half-life is longer than for methylphenidate, but dosing and effectiveness are similar.

This drug should not be used to combat fatigue or to replace rest in normal people.

Methylphenidate (Ritalin, Concerta, Metadate, Methylin, Daytrana)

Classification: CNS stimulant.

Used as: ADD and ADHD treatment; this is approved to be used as therapy in children 6 years of age and older. Long-term safety and efficacy in children has not been established. Some forms of methylphenidate are also approved to treat narcolepsy.[79]

Daily dosages above 60 mg are not recommended, with the notable exception that the FDA has approved Concerta in daily doses of up to 72 mg.

Unlabeled uses:

🜍 Depression in the medically ill elderly patients
  o Including stroke patients (Hayhow, Brockman, & Starkstein, 2014. pp. 227-240);

🜍 To treat neurobehavioral symptoms after traumatic brain injury (TBI)
  o There are mixed results with this use- all due to which area of the brain that has had damage (Johansson, Wentzel, Andréll, Odenstadt, Mannheimer, & Rönnbäck, 2013); and,

🜍 Improvement in pain control, to offset sedation, or both in patients receiving opiate therapy (Onishi, Biagioli, & Safranek, 2014; Bruera, Chadwick, Brenneis, Hanson, & MacDonald, 1987).

➢ And now, something to consider:

Dr. William A. Carlezon, Jr., Director of the behavioral genetics laboratory at McClean Hospital and associate professor at Harvard Medical School has reported that the use of Ritalin in children may increase the incidence of depression in later life. (Carlezon, Jr. & Konradi, 2004)

How does methylphenidate work?

It is thought to activate the brain stem arousal system (think about this for a minute- remember the "pain, pleasure, and rage" comment from earlier

---

[79] Several notes here:
1) Concerta, Metadate CD, and Ritalin LA are the only methylphenidate products approved to treat narcolepsy. That does not mean that one could not use Ritalin or Daytrana to treat narcolepsy just that those two products are not "officially" FDA approved.
2) Daytrana (the transdermal patch) is FDA approved only for ADHD.

116

and how each of those situations require that there be arousal) and affect the cerebral cortex.

Methylphenidate has its own "black box warning":

"Drug dependence: Give methylphenidate cautiously to emotionally unstable patients, such as those with a history of drug dependence or alcoholism, because such patients may increase dosage on their own initiative.

Chronic abuse can lead to marked tolerance and psychic dependence with varying degrees of abnormal behavior.

Frank psychotic episodes can occur, especially with parenteral abuse.

Careful supervision is required during drug withdrawal, because severe depression, as well as the effects of chronic overactivity, can be unmasked.

Long-term follow-up may be required because of the patient's basic personality disturbances."

Drug comparisons:

When compared to amphetamines, methylphenidate usually causes milder Central Nervous System (CNS) effects, and a greater impact on mental activities than on motor activities is observed.

This drug can cause physical and psychological (and social?) dependence when used for the indication of ADHD in children.

Drug excretion dynamics:

About 80% of the dose is metabolized to ritalinic acid, but this metabolism (and the subsequent half-life of methylphenidate- usually 1 to 3 hours) is similarly affected by hepatic impairment, then this drug is excreted by the kidneys at a rate of 67% for children (and, once again, this excretion percentage is decreased this time if there is renal impairment.)

Dexmethylphenidate (Focalin)

Classification: CNS stimulant.

Dexmethylphenidate is the *d*-threo enantiomeric isomer of racemic methylphenidate (which normally exists in the mixed enantiomeric state in the ratio of 50/50) - or, in plain English, this is the "right hand side" of methylphenidate (Ritalin and the others.)

Used as: ADHD treatment for children 6 years of age or older.

Drug comparisons:

Pretty much the same as methylphenidate.

Long-term use issues:

The effectiveness of the immediate release tablet form drug in treating clients for longer than 6 weeks has not been studied, nor has the use of the extended release capsules been studied for longer than 7 weeks.

Lisdexamfetamine dimesylate (Vyvanse)

This is one of the more interesting drugs in this book, and a favorite of the author. The reason? It does not work.

Allow an explanation!

Early on in this book, when discussing the benzodiazepine medications, the reader was presented with two medications that are "pro drugs"- drugs that have no therapeutic effect. Those two drugs must be turned into active medications within the body (using enzymes, another topic that has had quite a bit of discussion in this book!)

Lisdexamfetamine is rather like those other medications, in that lisdexamfetamine has no therapeutic effect. At all. That is, until the body uses enzymes and turns lisdexamfetamine into...dextroamphetamine (Dexedrine!)

Yep! Lisdexamfetamine is a lysine amino acid stuck onto a dextroamphetamine molecule. After ingestion, the body slices off the lysine amino acid[80] and the resulting product is dextroamphetamine.

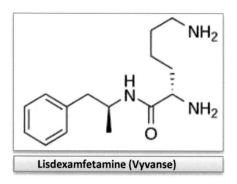

Lisdexamfetamine (Vyvanse)

So why have both dextroamphetamine and a drug that turns into dextroamphetamine? The answer is that people who take "straight" amphetamines (like amphetamine, dextroamphetamine, or methamphetamine) may have an improvement in attention (and have an effect on the pain response, the pleasure response, and the rage response- remember the Tiger?) but those same people may also get a "buzz"- the "pleasure" or "high." The drug levels decrease, and the people want to get that "high" again. This may lead to problems of abuse.

Lisdexamfetamine is thought to deliver a steady-state level of dextroamphetamine.

Graphically[81], see the difference in the concentrations of the individual medications in the bloodstream, and note that there is no "peak" with lisdexamfetamine.

---

[80] More trivia here, too! *L*-lysine (the left hand side of lysine) has been used to treat canker sores- also known as herpes zoster (Spar & Munóz, 2014)! Patients who take lisdexamfetamine get potential benefits for both shingles and ADD/ADHD; note well that the ongoing theme throughout this book- that infections and mental illnesses are intimately related!

[81] Again, this is for representation of the theory only! Note that the X-Axes and Y-Axes have the numbers "0" and "1." There is no such notation in the bloodstream of patients who take these medications. This is presented just to drive home a hypothetical point.

With dextroamphetamine (Dexedrine)

With lisdexamfetamine (Vyvanse)

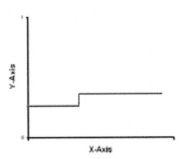

The idea is that if the medication may be altered so that there is less abuse potential, which is a good thing! And, because lisdexamfetamine is not "fun" it has little, if any, market value in the illicit drug trade.

One more thing about lisdexamfetamine and dextroamphetamine: these do not appear to "work" the same way for adults as they do for children- the clearance of these drugs decreases in adults ages 65-75 (26% in women and 10% in men).

Now, some "non-stimulating" ADHD medications...

Remember, "stimulants" cause the release of dopamine into the synaptic space (hence, "stimulate" the release).

🝠 **These next drugs are not thought to work on dopamine...**

Atomoxetine (Strattera)
Classification: Selective norepinephrine reuptake inhibitor (NRI).

This medication is a phenylpropanolamine derivative- and now that this has been stated, you, dear reader, may forget that! What one should remember is that atomoxetine is related to an old decongestant that was found in the old formulation of Dristan! Phenylpropanolamine is one atom (ONE ATOM!) different from amphetamine. Now does this mean that atomoxetine is related to amphetamine? Technically, no, but it is related to another chemical that is a derivative of amphetamine. Get it? ONE ATOM... "**atom**oxetine!"

Used as: Non-stimulating ADHD treatment. (Approved November 26, 2002.)

The safety of single doses over 120 mg and total daily doses in excess of 150 mg have not been systematically evaluated, and no benefits have been noted in any dose higher than 1.4 mg/kg/day. It is suggested that the dose not exceed that ¼ mg/kg/day level, or 100 mg a day, whichever is less (Spratto).

Drug comparisons:

Theoretically atomoxetine does not cause CNS excitation like the stimulants. Atomoxetine has a short half-life (5 hours), which can be extended by up to 3 more hours if given with food.

Dosage must be adjusted downward if there is hepatic insufficiency, and this medication has not been studied pharmacokinetically in children under age 6.

The professional circular recommends re-evaluating the client for therapeutic effects and presence/absence of side effects in 9 weeks for children and adolescents; 10 weeks for adults. Safety has not been evaluated beyond one year of use (Spratto).

Use caution when administering this drug to clients with narrow-angle glaucoma[82] due to mydriasis and those with cardiac conditions, and the use of this drug with rescue asthma medications like albuterol (Ventolin, Proventil) or levalbuterol (Xoponex) may significantly increase heart rate and blood pressure.

Weight loss must be monitored; growth does not seem to be affected, though; blood pressure must be monitored throughout the therapy. This medication has been reported to cause urinary retention.[83]

Guanfacine extended release (Intuniv).

The approximate retail price of guanfacine extended release at United States pharmacies is $549.60 per 100 tablets.

The "immediate release" guanfacine[84] sells at Wal-Mart for $4.00 for a 30-day supply of tablets, $10.00 for a 90-day supply.

How do these "work?"

Although the mechanism of action is unknown, Intuniv is thought to directly engage receptors found in the prefrontal cortex - an area of the brain that has been linked in preclinical research to ADHD.

Stimulation of the postsynaptic alpha 2 receptors is thought to strengthen working memory, reduce susceptibility to distraction, improve attention regulation, improve behavioral inhibition, and enhance impulse control.

What happens when those alpha 2 adrenergic receptors are stimulated?

By stimulating alpha 2 adrenergic receptors, guanfacine reduces sympathetic nerve impulses from the vasomotor center to the heart and blood vessels.

This results in a decrease in peripheral vascular resistance and a reduction in heart rate.

But, wait a minute!

Isn't this the exact OPPOSITE of what happens when we give someone a stimulant, or even Strattera?

The reason that this sounds just the opposite is, well, that it IS just the opposite!

But there is an explanation!

---

[82] This, too, should make sense to readers of this book. Recall that atom**oxetine** (Strattera) is chemically related to par**oxetine** (Paxil, Pexeva, Brisdelle), flu**oxetine** (Prozac, Sarafem), dul**oxetine** (Cymbalta), and even vorti**oxetine** (Brintellix)- and all these are thought to "work" on norepinephrine and serotonin...just like the tricyclic and tetracyclic antidepressants are thought to "work" on the" tiger chemical" (norepinephrine) and maybe serotonin. The TCAs (and others listed above) may have an effect on the iris sphincter, which is innervated by the parasympathetic nervous system and the iris dilator innervated by the sympathetic nervous system. Using drug that affect the parasympathetic or sympathetic system may cause problems in patients with glaucoma.

[83] That urinary retention side effect possibility should make sense to you, gentle reader, by now. Remember that the first tricyclic antidepressant- imipramine (Tofranil) has a use that is not officially FDA approved- to treat bedwetting! And the TCAs are thought to work on...norepinephrine, just like atomoxetine!

[84] The brand name of guanfacine immediate release is Tenex.

121

YIN AND YANG!

In each of us, there exists the nervous system:

☯ Part of this is known as the "sympathetic" nervous system

☯ Part is known as the "parasympathetic" nervous system

They "offset" each other, existing in an exquisite balance (most of the time). And if the sympathetic and parasympathetic nervous systems are "out of balance" there is thought to be disease...just like if Yin and Yang are "out of balance."

With either guanfacine (Intuniv) or the sister drug clonidine (Kapvay, discussed below) should the patient experience any of the following side effects the prescribing physician should be notified as soon as possible:

Fainting	Shortness of breath or difficulty breathing
Swollen feet, ankles, or wrists	Fast, pounding, or irregular heartbeat

Clonidine (Catapres, Kapvay, and several others)

Classification: alpha adrenergic agonist (remember, agonists "increase"). This extended-release form was approved by the FDA as an "add-on" treatment (with stimulant medications) and as a monotherapy for ADHD.

Uses (official FDA and non-official FDA approvals):

Antidysmenorrheal	Antihypertensive
To treat tachycardia	Stress
Sleep disorders	Borderline personality disorder
Anxiety disorders	Post-operative and intractable pain relief
Used as an epidural to treat pain during heart attack	As a premedication before surgery or other medical procedures
Menopausal syndrome therapy adjunct	Has been used in treating autism
Opioid, alcohol, and nicotine withdrawal syndrome suppressant	Restless legs syndrome
Rosacea	To treat diabetic neuropathy
To treat migraines	Vascular headache prophylactic
For treatment of the very rare instances of dexmedetomidine (an anæsthetic used in ICUs and by anæsthesiologists and, no kidding, in veterinary medicine) withdrawal	

Clonidine has an "orphan drug" status as of 1989:

"...for continuous epidural administration as adjunctive therapy with intraspinal opiates for pain in cancer patients tolerant or unresponsive to intraspinal opiates." (United States Food and Drug Administration, 2013)

Odd that it is used for narcotic withdrawal, eh?

Now the antipsychotics

This book will "lump" these medications together in the following format:

"Typical" antipsychotics **"Atypical" antipsychotics**

There is a reason for this "lumping together"- ALL antipsychotic medications are thought to "work" by blocking dopamine at the dopamine D2 receptors.

ALL OF THE ANTIPSYCHOTIC MEDICATIONS!

The "Typical" antipsychotics

This class of medications might be better named "Traditional" antipsychotics or the "Conventional" antipsychotic medications.

Just a discussion on phenothiazines[85], as a sub-class, in general:

- ☧ Never re-expose clients to phenothiazine agents if they developed jaundice;
- ☧ The use of any of the phenothiazine drugs in infants younger than 1 year of age may be a factor in SIDS (Kessler, Harrison, & Hagemann, 2010);
- ☧ Discontinue the use of phenothiazines at least 48 hours prior to myelography due to seizure risk;
- ☧ All phenothiazines must be used carefully in patients with respiratory impairments- "Silent pneumonia" may develop; and,
- ☧ All phenothiazines may carry a risk of causing adynamic ileus.

Chlorpromazine (Thorazine)

Classification: Antipsychotic; Aliphatic phenothiazine.

While the "exact mechanism of action" is not understood, it is believed that this drug may exert its effect due to post-synaptic block of either/or adrenergic and dopaminergic receptor sites. Additional theories include acting to decrease the excitability of the neuronal membranes or by metabolic inhibition of oxylated phosphorylation.

Used as: Antipsychotic.

This medication is also approved for:

As adjunctive treatment for tetanus	To treat intractable hiccoughs	For acute intermittent porphyria
For treatment of mania	☧	Nausea and vomiting
For the treatment of severe behavioral problems in children 1 to 12 years of age	For relief of presurgical restlessness and apprehension	

And some unapproved uses:

For treatment of PCP-induced psychosis	For treatment of migraine headaches

Drug comparisons:

With other agents available in the United States, this drug is used less often than in previous years. Chlorpromazine produces more sedation and

---

[85] The reader will recall that the "phenothiazine" medications were discussed early on in this book when the history of psychopharmacological agents was addressed. Remember the quest for quinine that lead to the blue dyes (methylene blue and summer blue)?

hypotension than haloperidol or other agents. Therapeutically it may be beneficial to "use" the sedation side effect if clinically indicated. DO understand that sometimes the other side effects outweigh the benefits of this sedation, however. Hypotension may be significant.

℞ Add to this the sedation and the client may be at significant risk for falls.

There is a risk of Tardive Dyskinesia (more on this later in the book.)

The occurrence of extrapyramidal symptoms (Parkinson's Disease-like hand shakiness and gait disturbances) was said to occur less frequently with the newer "atypical" antipsychotic medications than with the more "potent" antipsychotics, such as chlorpromazine (probably due to the inherency of chlorpromazine causing anticholinergic side effects, but that anticholinergic side effect may be problematic.) Chlorpromazine may cause skin pigmentation changes or photosensitivity.

And now a discussion on antipsychotic medication comparisons:

When comparing to the newer, "atypical" antipsychotics, some have said that Thorazine (and others in this class of "typical" antipsychotics) are less effective overall (especially in treating the "negative" symptoms) in treatment-resistant clients. But when focusing on efficacy of antipsychotic medications in general, the atypical antipsychotics have been said to be more effective than the older antipsychotic drugs against "negative" symptoms of schizophrenia, including:

1. Emotional flatness or lack of expression;
2. Inability to start or follow through with activities; and,
3. Speech that is brief and lacks content, and lack of pleasure or interest in life

But overall, **no evidence** suggested that any of the atypical antipsychotics had a special effect on either the negative or "positive" symptoms (which include delusions and hallucinations) that occur because the patient has lost touch with reality in important ways[86].

Perphenazine (Trilafon)
Classification: Antipsychotic; Phenothiazine; Piperazine.
A true "tranquilizer," this drug acts at all levels of the CNS.
The exact mechanism of action is not known[87].
Used as: Antipsychotic; Antiemetic.
Unlabeled use: To treat intractable hiccoughs (IV only).
Drug comparisons:
Perphenazine is available as an injection as well as in an oral dosage form.

"The old standby," this drug works!

Even though this drug "works", it does have a risk of Tardive Dyskinesia (TD), and Extrapyramidal Symptoms (EPS) are not uncommon. There is a low

---

[86] This will also be discussed a little more in detail in a few pages.
[87] The reader has noticed that this concept, too, is an ongoing theme throughout this book.

incidence of ocular changes (this is less anticholinergic than some other antipsychotic medications) but one may encounter some depositing of particulate matter in the lens and cornea (which may progress in more severe cases to a "star-shaped" lenticular opacity. Some cases of ocular keratopathy and even pigmentary retinopathy (yes, perphenazine may change the color of a patient's eye!)[88] have been reported with the use of this medication.

Blood dyscrasias (changes in the blood cells) do not routinely occur with perphenazine, and there is less incidence of jaundice than with some of the other medications used in this class, which means less concern about liver involvement. Perphenazine has only moderate hypotensive and sedative effects- but note that the IM form appears to cause more hypotension than the oral form.

Pimozide (Orap)

Classification: Antipsychotic; a diphenylbutylpiperidine.[89]

Pimozide is thought to reduce hallucinations and delusions through blockade of dopamine D_2 receptors[90] in the mesolimbic area of the brain as well as through blockade in the nigrostriatal pathway (which accounts for the EPS- the nigrostriatal pathway is where Parkinson's Disease is thought to occur). This medication is a high-affinity central dopamine-2 (D_2) receptor antagonist, with the primary receptor sites being affected being postsynaptic.

Used as: Ah, this is where it gets a little strange! This antipsychotic medication is not used for psychosis! Nope! It is used as a Tourette's Disorder drug treatment for children older than twelve years of age and adults! But, this drug is NOT to be used to treat drug-induced motor or phonic tics, such as those caused by stimulants.

This medication is used "off-label" to treat schizophrenia in children, and has been reported to be better for treating of monosymptomatic hypochondriasis (Riding & Munro, 1975) as well as delusional disorder, paranoid personality disorder (Riding), and- here is one that is odd- delusions caused by parasitosis[91] (van Vloten, 2003). Does the reader think that use is odd? How about the fact that the medication Pimozide has been suggested to be effective against *Listeria monocytogenes*[92]? (Lieberman & Higgins, 2009)

This drug has been around a while, being approved by the FDA July 31, 1984.

Drug comparisons:

Pimozide is rather on its own, being neither a typical nor an atypical antipsychotic. One might even consider this to be a "neuroleptic" agent.

---

[88] Understand that this is not the only antipsychotic medication that may, as opposed to the Country Western song, not only make one's "brown eyes blue" but could cause the opposite result!

[89] Goodness, do not pharmacists like to use fancy sounding chemical names?

[90] Remember well that **ALL** antipsychotic medications are thought to "work" by blocking dopamine at the dopamine D2 receptors.

[91] O.K., one might make an argument that parasitosis is also an "infection"- going back to the theme of the intimate relationship between psychopharmacology and infection (infestation.)

[92] See the footnote above- the extremely interesting interrelationship of infections and mental health!

Pimozide may be cardiotoxic; for this reason, this drug must be used very carefully with other QTc prolonging agents.

There are other First Generation Antipsychotic (FGA) medications, such as Vesprin, Haldol, Thorazine, Mellaril, Prolixin, and Stelazine, several of which are no longer marketed, and some of which are only available generically. But keeping to the focus of this book being only a Primer, these other FGAs will not be addressed.

The "Atypical" antipsychotics

There is not a definition as to what makes a drug an atypical antipsychotic- this is a phrase from history. When the first atypical antipsychotic (clozapine [Clozaril]) was being studied one of the researchers noted that this medication did not cause any extrapyramidal (EPS) symptoms- that "hand shaky" thing. The researcher wrote: "This antipsychotic is atypical from others currently on the market (Weiden, 2007)."

The name stuck.

The pharmaceutical companies marketing these atypical antipsychotics (these will be called "the atypicals" from now on in this book) suggested that these medications share a commonality in that these drugs have the ability to produce a therapeutic effect (antipsychotic effect) with few or no acutely occurring extrapyramidal side effects (EPS).

When the marketing of these atypicals began, the medical community and the public were told that, as a rule, there are also no significant tardive dyskinesias attributable to the employment of these medications. Tardive dyskinesia was a problem sometimes seen when the older antipsychotic medications, like chlorpromazine (Thorazine), thioridazine (Mellaril), and others were taken by patients.

Likewise, marketing suggested that when the atypical antipsychotic medications were taken by patients, one did not usually see an effect on serum prolactin. The older, First Generation (FGA) antipsychotic medications were known to rarely cause breast enlargement in both genders; both genders could begin producing breast milk.

Understand that the use of atypical antipsychotic medications indeed may result in tardive dyskinesia, extrapyramidal symptoms, and hyperprolactinemia (Ajmal, Joffe, & Nachtigall, 2014; Friedman, 2012).

While these medications may have one or more of these benefits to therapeutic choice, the only one drug that fits the previous criteria is the prototype: Clozapine (Clozaril). Clozapine may cause some serious, sometimes life-threatening, changes to the white blood cells of patients.

Are these newer antipsychotic medications more effective?

British physicians, who were developing guidelines, used meta-analysis to systematically review randomized controlled clinical trials for treating schizophrenia with this group of new drugs called "atypical antipsychotics." This research found no clear evidence that "atypical antipsychotics" are more effective or better tolerated than older, conventional antipsychotics. The recommendation from this extensive effort--published in the December 2, 2000, British Medical Journal (BMJ)--was that the older, conventional antipsychotics should be tried first (Geddes, Freemantle, Harrison, & Bebbington, 2000).

The CATIE report...

There is quite a bit of controversy over this study, which focused on comparisons between the atypical, Second Generation Antipsychotics and the older, traditional First Generation Antipsychotics:

"A landmark government-financed study that compared drugs used to treat schizophrenia has confirmed what many psychiatrists long suspected-
- Newer drugs that are highly promoted and widely prescribed offer few- if any- benefits over older medications that sell for a fraction of the cost. From that study, almost 75% of the patients taking the newer drugs stopped taking them because of discomfort or specific side effects (Carey, 2005).*"*

Specific reasons for stopping the individual SGA medication included:
- The drug that the patients was taking was not effective;
- The patient could not tolerate the specific test drug; and,
- There were significant side effects like sleeplessness, tremors, stiffness, and weight gain.

This report was published in the *New England Journal of Medicine* on September 22, 2005 (Lieberman, Stroup, McEvoy, Swartz, Rosenheck, Perkins, Keefe, Davis, Davis, Lebowitz, Severe, & Hsiao).[93]

There are some concerns about atypical antipsychotic drugs and stroke.

New expert advice issued March 5, 2004 recommends that two atypical antipsychotic drugs, risperidone and olanzapine, should not be used to treat behavioural problems in older patients with dementia. The Committee on Safety of Medicines (CSM) has reviewed the data for risperidone and olanzapine, and reported that the evidence showed that there is a three-fold increase in the risk of stroke for risperidone when used in older patients with dementia with a similar risk with olanzapine (Medicines and Healthcare Products Regulatory Agency, 2004).

There is more on the use of these drugs with the elderly-
WASHINGTON, April 11, 2005
The US Food and Drug Administration (FDA) on Monday ordered new warnings on antipsychotic drugs because they have

---

[93] The reader of this book should understand that the CATIE study and the 2000 study from England are not intended to be seen as attacks on the use of the atypical antipsychotic medications, the SGAs. No, indeed, these reports are mentioned solely to reinforce the fact that clinicians will use whatever medications are in the available armamentarium to treat patients with schizophrenia (and do not forget, these SGAs are also used to treat bipolar disorder)- but sometimes there is little difference in effectiveness, side effects, and compliance with therapy. These two references, the Geddes study from Great Britain and the CATIE study, are presented to reinforce that there are significant differences in costs of these medications. When Benedict Carey reported the results of the CATIE study in the 2005 *USA Today* article, the costs of these medications- at equipotent dosing- were as follows: "In the doses used in the study, a month's supply of perphenazine costs about $60, compared with $520 for Zyprexa, $450 for Seroquel, $250 for Risperdal and $290 for Geodon (Carey, 2005)."

been in studies linked to higher mortality among the old people who take the drug for dementia-related symptoms.

The agency said it is asking manufacturers of atypical antipsychotic drugs to add to their labeling a boxed warning noting the risks and that the drugs are not approved to treat symptoms of dementia in the elderly.

The drugs are approved for treating schizophrenia and mania.

They include Bristol-Myers Squibb and Otsuka America Pharmaceutical's Abilify, Eli Lilly and Co.'s Zyprexa, AstraZeneca Pharmaceuticals LP's Seroquel, Johnson and Johnson's Risperdal, Novartis AG's Clozaril and Pfizer Inc.'s Geodon.

The warning order also affects Eli Lilly and Co.'s Symbyax, which is approved for treatment of depressive episodes associated with bipolar disorder.

Patients should consult their doctors before taking the drugs for dementia-related symptoms, said the FDA.

An analysis of 17 studies involving four drugs showed the rate of death for the elderly patients with dementia who took the drugs was about 1.6 to 1.7 times that for placebo users.

The FDA said the causes of death varied, but most seemed to be heart-related or from infections.

The four atypical antipsychotics tested cover all the three classes of the drug based on their chemical structure, according to the agency (China View, 2005).

There are more concerns about the use of atypical antipsychotics

On September 1, 2004, the FDA made the following announcement:

The FDA recommends that all patients treated with atypical antipsychotics be monitored for symptoms of hyperglycemia and undergo fasting blood glucose testing upon presentation. Patients diagnosed with diabetes mellitus should be monitored regularly for loss of glucose control.

Patients with traditional diabetes mellitus risk factors should undergo fasting blood glucose testing at initiation of treatment with atypical antipsychotics (FDA Patient Safety News, 2004.)

The above warning is notable in that one will see that this applies not just to individuals with psychosis, but rather ALL patients treated with atypical antipsychotic medications, regardless of the diagnosis. Now, parallel the warning about hyperglycemia, and consider that some patients, when pregnant, do experience:

- Breast enlargement (indeed, hyperprolactinemia and gynecomastia are sometimes side effects of antipsychotic medications)
- Difficulty in controlling blood sugar (gestational diabetes)

130

Add to this the concept that some patients with diabetes are more prone to risk factors that could lead to an early death, notably, heart attack, infection, and stroke.

Now review the fact that the FDA says not to use these medications in elderly patients with dementia because of a greater risk of death due to...heart attack, infection, and stroke. Even though the FDA says not to use these medications in elderly patients with dementia, almost one out of every four patients in nursing homes in the United States are receiving one – or more!- of these medications (Briesacher, Tija, Field, Peterson, & Gurwitz, 2013.)

Generic name (Brand Name)	% of total prescriptions	Atypical or Conventional
Quetiapine (Seroquel)	31.1	Atypical
Risperidone (Risperdal)	24.4	Atypical
Olanzapine (Zyprexa)	13.1	Atypical
Haloperidol (Haldol)	9.2	Conventional
Clozapine (Clozaril)	5.3	Atypical
Ziprasidone (Geodon)	3.2	Atypical
Chlorpromazine (Thorazine)	1.5	Conventional
Fluphenazine (Trilafon)	1.3	Conventional
All others[94]	2.9	Mixture of both

Table modified heavily from Briesacher et al., 2013. This chart represents the most commonly prescribed antipsychotic medications in nursing homes from September 2009 through October 2010.

Now on to some (not all, remember, this is a Primer) of the Atypical Antipsychotic medications!

Aripiprazole (Abilify)

Classification: Atypical antipsychotic; Psychotropic; a quinolone derivative.

This medication has been reported to have an affinity for several neurotransmitter receptors. It is said to have partial AGONISTIC (remember, "turns on the cell" from the beginning of this book on page 16) activity at D_2 and $5\text{-}HT_1$, but potent ANTAGONISM ("turns off") at $5\text{-}HT_{2a}$ receptors. Why is this topic- that aripiprazole potentially affects multiple sites of neurotransmitter activity- in this book? Well, this means that theoretically aripiprazole may also have some activity at some of the same receptors as the SSRIs without causing as much cognitive impairment. It is for this specific reason- potential serotonergic activity- that the FDA has approved aripiprazole

---

[94] Paliperidone (Invega, atypical); perphenazine (Trilafon, conventional); thiothixene (Navane, conventional); loxapine (Loxitane, conventional); trifluoperazine (Stelazine, conventional); combination of olanzapine and fluoxetine (Symbyax, atypical plus SSRI); asenapine (Saphris, atypical); iloperidone (Fanapt, atypical); molindone (Moban, conventional); pimozide (Orap, conventional); mesoridazine (Serentil, conventional.)

not only as an antipsychotic medication, but also is approved to treat bipolar disorder (manic or mixed episode as well as for acute mania), as an adjunct (add-on) therapy when a patient is taking antidepressants and not getting the desired therapeutic improvement, and to treat the irritability associated with autism[95].

Drug comparisons:

There still may be a risk of neuroleptic malignant syndrome (NMS), and aripiprazole has been suggested to rarely cause orthostatic hypotension. This medication must be used in caution with clients having a history of seizure. This medication has been reported to be pretty good for the melancholic client, the anhedonic patient, or the unmotivated client whose condition may worsen with the use of SSRIs.

Olanzapine (Zyprexa)

Classification: Atypical antipsychotic.

Note well! Olazapine is "chemically classified" as a member of the thieno**benzodiazepine** class of drugs!

Sedation may be notable (and, possibly, clinically indicated)

Pharmacological effect:

This medication is thought to binds to dopamine and serotonin receptors, and may interfere with histaminergic, cholinergic, and adrenergic receptors. Sounds a little like the other benzodiazepine medications that are thought to work on GABA ("the brakes of the brain"), does it not?

In addition to FDA approval as an antipsychotic medication, other official FDA approvals include use for:

- ℞ Treatment as a monotherapy for acute mixed or manic episodes of Bipolar I disorder;
- ℞ Treatment, in conjunction with lithium, for short-term treatment of acute mixed or manic episodes associated with Bipolar I disorder;
- ℞ Treatment, in conjunction with fluoxetine (Prozac) to treat depressive episodes associated with Bipolar I disorder (Eli Lilly marketed the combination drug Symbyax, which contains both olanzapine and fluoxetine- the combination is now also available generically);
- ℞ Treatment, again in combination with fluoxetine (Prozac) for patients with treatment-resistant depression (major depressive disorder); and;
- ℞ As a treatment for pediatric schizophrenia and Bipolar I disorder- but only "...after a thorough diagnostic evaluation along with careful consideration of the risks associated with drug treatment." (Spratto).
- ℞ The intramuscular injection form of olanzapine is approved to treat agitation associated with schizophrenia and Bipolar I disorder, and

---

[95] This concept, that aripiprazole might be of benefit for "irritability" should make sense, as many times in pediatric patients one of the most striking clinical presentations of depression is...irritability.

the intramuscular injection form of olanzapine pamoate (Zyprexa Relprevv)[96] is approved for the treatment of schizophrenia.

Investigationally, this medication is being studied as a treatment of obsessive-compulsive disorder (OCD) that is refractory to SSRIs; for delusional parasitosis (remember that this was discussed as a treatment for pimozide (ORAP) earlier in this book on page 121); stuttering; Tourette's in adults, adolescents, and children; and, for the psychosis and agitation in patients with dementia and Alzheimer's (although the FDA has issued specific warnings at this time to NOT use atypical antipsychotic medications for agitation in these clients.)

Risperidone (Risperdal)

Classification: Atypical antipsychotic; Benzisoxazole derivative.

This medication shows antagonistic activity for both dopamine type 2 and serotonin type 2.

Risperdal has the first water-based antipsychotic injection in the US, known as Risperdal Consta. Risperdal Consta is a saline-based solution and is approved in the U.S. and Europe'; this formulation is associated with less pain upon injection that the old, oil-based antipsychotics, and is given once every two weeks.

Used as:

Acute and maintenance treatment of schizophrenia in adults	Treatment of adolescent (ages 13-17 years) schizophrenia
For the short-term treatment, as a monotherapy, of acute manic or mixed Bipolar I disorder episodes	
In combination with lithium or valproate (Depakote) for the adults short-term treatment of acute mixed or manic Bipolar I episodes	
For the irritability associated with autistic disorder in children and adolescents (the age range here is between five and sixteen years of age); this includes symptoms of aggression toward others, temper tantrums, deliberate SIB (self-injurious behaviors), and "quickly changing moods."[97]	

Risperidone has been studied for treatment refractory OCD (when SSRIs do not "work"), stuttering, Tourette's syndrome, and the psychosis and/or agitation sometimes seen in dementia and Alzheimer's Disease. REMEMBER-THERE IS AN FDA WARNING TO NOT USE THE ATYPICAL ANTIPSYCHOTIC MEDICATIONS IN THE ELDERLY PATIENT WITH DEMENTIA!

---

[96] Here is a weird one- if a patient received the intramuscular (IM) injection of olanzapine pamoate, there is a risk of fatal heart consequences. The FDA requires that clinicians who administer the IM olanzapine pamoate have ready access to emergency response service, and that the patients who receive must be monitored for at least three hours. This medication is available only through a restricted distribution program, and the patients, the health care provider, the health care facility, and pharmacy all be enrolled in that program. The FDA is also investigating two patient deaths, where the deaths occurred 3-4 days after receiving "...an appropriate dose of the drug (FDA, 2013)."

[97] That "quickly changing mood" approval will have profound clinical implications for children diagnosed under the DSM-5 with the new condition: "Disruptive Mood Dysregulation Disorder." The reader of this book is directed to the DSM-5 (APA).

Drug comparisons:

This medication was marketed to the public as "the most often used drug in its class."[98]

This drug seems to have more of an effect on prolactin levels than other atypical agents, so it is important to watch for breast enlargement in all patients, regardless of gender. Additionally, risperidone may have a "troublesome" side effect of causing an antiemetic effect- which could obscure signs and symptoms of overdosage or physical conditions, like intestinal obstruction, Reye's Syndrome, or a brain tumor.

There are more possible side effects with risperidone (Risperdal):

- Some reports of ECG irregularities
- Priapism has been reported
- There is still a possibility of TD

As mentioned at the beginning of this section dealing with atypical antipsychotic medications, the SGAs, there are many more. But remember that ALL antipsychotic medications- First Generation and Second Generation- are thought to "work" by blocking dopamine activity at dopamine D2 receptors.

For that reason, here is a list **only** of the second generation antipsychotic medications currently available in the United States- if you know how one "works" you know how all of them "work." Remember, too, that some of these SGAs are "thought" to work on other neurotransmitters, like serotonin, norepinephrine, etc.:

Aripiprazole (marketed as Abilify)	Asenapine Maleate (marketed as Saphris)	Clozapine (marketed as Clozaril)
Iloperidone (marketed as Fanapt)	Lurasidone (marketed as Latuda)	Olanzapine (marketed as Zyprexa)
Olanzapine/Fluoxetine (marketed as Symbyax)	Paliperidone (marketed as Invega)	Quetiapine (marketed as Seroquel)
Risperidone (marketed as Risperdal)	Ziprasidone (marketed as Geodon)	

Lurasidone (Latuda) was being marketed as being an atypical antipsychotic that did not have a problem with weight gain. The manufacturer is no longer making that marketing claim. Lurasidone is now approved not only to treat schizophrenia, but also to treat the depressive episodes of Bipolar I disorder (as is Symbyax.)

Paliperidone (Invega) is the active metabolite of risperidone (Risperdal) and has FDA approvals for acute and maintenance treatment of schizophrenia in adults and adolescents (between the ages of 12-17) and as an acute treatment as monotherapy (or with mood stabilizers) for schizoaffective disorder.

---

[98] One could make an entire book just on pharmacy marketing. Understand that this author is not deriding marketing, or pharmacy manufacturers. Pharmacy companies have one job, and one job only- to return dividends to shareholders. If you, Gentle Reader, have mutual funds in your retirement program, then you "own" a pharmacy company. Several, probably, as mutual funds are big "baskets of stocks"- and pharmacy companies are very profitable ventures.

Quetiapine (Seroquel) is approved by the FDA as an "add-on" treatment for patients who are taking antidepressants and not getting the therapeutic results expected, just like Abilify is approved as an "add-on." The reason for quetiapine (Seroquel) getting that approval is that quetiapine is thought to have some effect on norepinephrine (the "Tiger Chemical" from the beginning of this book.) Remember, when one is being chased by a tiger, one is not depressed! Additionally, quetiapine (Seroquel) is approved by the FDA as a treatment for the depressive episodes of Bipolar I disorder either as monotherapy or with lithium or divalproate (Depakote), rather like olanzapine (Zyprexa) is approved. Quetiapine (Seroquel) is being used- sometimes even in pediatric patients- as a somnotic (sleep inducer.) This author feels that if one is going to use quetiapine as a sleeping medication, one might as well prescribe chlorpromazine (Thorazine). Of interest is that quetiapine is becoming a drug of abuse! Opioid-dependent patients who are taking the combination drug buprenorphine and naloxone (Suboxone) have been told that those patients cannot abuse the product, as Suboxone is a combination opioid agonist (turns on the receptor-this is the buprenorphine) and antagonist (blocks the receptor- this is the naloxone.) The idea is that a patient trying to get a "heroin high" by using Suboxone will go into immediate withdrawal symptoms because of the naloxone. Well, substance abusers found out that by taking quetiapine (Seroquel) that the withdrawal from an overdose of Suboxone can be "softened". Quetiapine even has street names among drug abusers- "Susie Q", "Quell","Q-Ball", and "Baby Heroin."

Finishing the SGAs, look at the similarities of the generic names:

Lurasi**DONE**	Ziprasi**DONE**
Iloperi**DONE**	Paliperi**DONE**
Even haloperi**DONE** (Haldol)[99]	

That means, Dear Reader, that these all "share" part of the chemical structure!

And with that, it is the hope that psychopharmacology is now a little more understandable. Remember: Look at what the body does "naturally" and use medicine- psychopharmacology- to either increase or decrease that response!

---

[99] The astute Reader in the United States will say: "Hey, wait a minute! The generic name of Haldol is haloperidol!" That is correct...in the United States! Overseas, Haldol is known generically as "haloperidone" due to the presence of a ketone in the chemical structure. The purpose of including haloperidone in this table is to reaffirm that many of these medications "share" components of the chemical structure.

111th United States Congress. (2014. February 5). Patient Protection and Affordable Care Act, P.L. 111-148. Retrieved from http://wikipedia.org/wiki/Patient_Protection_and_Affordable_Care_Act

ABC News (2000, September 14). Tyson: Drug Stops Me From Killing You! [Network Broadcast]. Retrieved from http://abcnews.go.com/Sports/story?id=100564

Adam, K., & Oswald, I. (1993, May). Triazolam: Unpublished manufacturers research unfavourable. *British Medical Journal, 306*(6890), 1475-1476.

Ajmal, A., Joffe, H., & Nachtigall, L. B. (2014, January-February). Psychotropic-induced hyperprolactinemia: a clinical review. *Psychosomatics, 55*(1), 29-36.

American Psychiatric Association (2013). *Diagnostic and Statistical Manual of Mental Disorders, Fifth Edition*. Arlington, Virginia: American Psychiatric Association.

Anderson, I. M. (2000). Selective serotonin reuptake inhibitors versus tricyclic antidepressants: a meta-analysis of efficacy and tolerability. *Journal of Affective Disorders, 58*(1), 19-36.

Anderson, J. A., Mizgalewicz, A., & Illes, J. (2013). Triangulating perspectives on functional neuroimaging for disorders of mental health. *BMC Psychiatry, 13(*208), 1-11. doi: 10.1186-1471-244X-13-208

Banov, M. D. (2010). *Taking antidepressants: Your comprehensive guide to starting, staying on, and safely quitting.* North Branch, MN: Sunrise Silver Press.

Benfield, D. G., & Kelley, C. S. (2010). *Prescription drugs in pregnancy.* Ashland, OH: AtlasBooks.

Briesacher, B. A., Tija, J., Field, T., Peterson, D., & Gurwitz, J.H. (2013, February 6). Antipsychotic use among nursing home residents. *The Journal of the American Medical Association, 309*(5), 440-442. Doi.10.1001/jama.2012.211266

Bruera, E., Chadwick, S., Brenneis, C., Hanson, J., & MacDonald, R. N. (1987, January). Methylphenidate associated with narcotics for the treatment of cancer pain. *Cancer Treatment Reports, 71*(1), 67-70.

Brunt, T. M., Koeter, M. W., Hertoghs, N., van Noorden, M. S., & van den Brink, W. (2013, August). Sociodemographic and substance use characteristics of gamma hydroxybutyrate (GHB) dependent inpatients and associations with dependence severity. *Drug and Alcohol Dependence, 131*(3), 316-319.

Canadian Adverse Drug Reaction Monitoring Program (CADRMP), Marketed Health Products Directorate, HEALTH CANADA. (2006, May). Health Canada Issued Important Safety Information on ADHD Drugs. Retrieved from http://www.psychrights.org/research/Digest/ADHD/adhd-tdah_medic-hpc-cps_ehealthcanada.pdf

Carey, B. (2005, September 20). Little difference found in schizophrenia drugs. Retrieved from http://nytimes.com/2005/09/20/health/psychology/20drug.htm

Carlezon, Jr., W. A., & Konradi, C. (2004). Understanding the neurobiological consequences of early exposure to psychotropic drugs: linking behavior with molecules. *Neuropharmacology, 47*, Supplement 1, 47-60.

Carrey, N., & Virani, A. (2003, November). Suicidal ideation reports from pediatric trials for paroxetine and venlafaxine. *Canadian Child and Adolescent Psychiatric Review, 12*(4), 101-102.

Center for Substance Abuse Research- University of Maryland. (2013, Oct 29). Amphetamines. Retrieved from http://www.cesar.umd.edu/cesar/drugs/amphetamines.asp

Centers for Disease Control. (2008, October 22). Depression Hurts. So Do Antidepressants. Retrieved from *http://antidepression.wordpress.com/2008/10/22/history-of-antidepressants/*

Centers for Disease Control. (2008, October 22). History of Antidepressants. Retrieved from *http://antidepression.wordpress.com/2008/10/22/history-of-antidepressants*

China View. (2005, April 12). FDA orders warning on use of antipsychotic drugs by elderly. Retrieved from *http://news.xinhuanet.com/English/2005-04/12/content_2828182.htm*.

Christensen, J., Grønborg, T. K., Sorensen, M. J., Schendel, D., Parner, E. T., Pedersen, L. H., & Vestergaard, M. (2013, April 24). Prenatal valproate exposure and risk of autism spectrum disorders and childhood autism. *Journal of the American Medical Association, 309*(16), 1698-1703.

Ciarleglio, C. M., Axley, J. C., Strauss, B. R., Gamble, K. L., & McMahon, D. G. (2011). Perinatal photoperiod imprints the circadian clock. *Nature Neuroscience, 14*, 25-27. doi: 10.1038.nn.2699

Coplan, J. D., Andrews, M. W., Rosenblum, L. A., Owens, M. J., Friedman, S., Gorman, J. M., & Nemeroff, C. B. (1996, February). Persistent elevations of cerebrospinal fluid concentrations of corticotrophin-releasing factor in adult nonhuman primates exposed to early life stressors: Implications for the pathophysiology of mood and anxiety disorders. *Proceeds of the National Academy of Sciences, USA, 93*(4), 1619-1623.

Croen, L. A., Grether, J. K., Yoshida, C. K., Odouli, R., & Hendrick, V. (2014, July). Antidepressant use during pregnancy and childhood autism spectrum disorders. *Archives of General Psychiatry, 68*(11), 1104-1112. doi:10.1001/archgenpsychiatry.2011.73

Dauvilliers, Y., Carlander, B., Molinari, N., Desautels, A., Okum, M., Tafti, M., Montplaisir, J., Mignot, E., & Billiard, M. (2003, September). Month of birth as a risk factor for narcolepsy. *Sleep, 26*(6), 663-665.

Davies, G., Welham, J., Chant, D., Torrey, E. F., & McGrath, J. (2003). A systematic review and meta-analysis of northern hemisphere season of birth studies in schizophrenia. *Schizophrenia Bulletin, 29*(3), 587-593.

Department of Health & Human Services, Food and Drug Administration. (2012, June 25). Equetro Letter- Food and Drug Administration. Retrieved from http://www.fda.gov.downloads/Drugs/GuidanceComplianceRegulatoryInformation/Enforcement/Activit esbyFDA/WarningLettersandNoticesofViolationLetterstoPharmaceuticalCompanies/UCM313060.pdf

Donaldson, M., Gizzarelli, G, & Chanpong, B. (2007, Fall). Oral sedation: a primer on anxiolysis for the adult patient. *Anesthesia Progress, 54*(3): 118-129.

Drugs.com. (2005, February). Health Canada suspends market authorization of Adderall XR for ADHD in children. Retrieved from http://www.drugs.com/news/health-canada-suspends-market-authorization-adderall-xr-adhd-children-3601.html

Ensminger, P. A. (2001). *Life under the sun*. Harrisburg, PA: R.R. Donnelley & Sons.

Escitalopram (Lexapro) for depression. (2002, September 30). *The Medical Letter, 44*(1170), 83-4.

Express Scripts, Gold Standard, An Elsevier Company. (2009, July 8). DrugDigest.org: Desoxyn Tablets. Retrieved from http://www.drugdigest.org

FDA Patient Safety News: Show #28. (June 2004). Warning about hyperglycemia and atypical antipsychotic drugs. Retrieved from http://www.accessdata.fda.gov/psn/printer.cfm?id-229.

FindLaw for Legal Professionals. (2008, March 26). Off-label Provisions of the Food and Drug Modernization Act Found Unconstitutional. Retrieved from http://corporatefindlaw.com/litigation-disputes/off-label-provisions-of-the-food-and-drug-modernization-act-found.html

Foster, R., & Kreitzman, L. (2010). *Seasons of life: The biological rhythms that enable living things to thrive and survive*. London: Profile Books, LTD.

Friedman, R. A. (2012, September 24). A call for caution on antipsychotic drugs. *The New York Times*, D6.

Geddes, J., Freemantle, N., Harrison, P., & Bebbington, P. (2000, December 2). Atypical antipsychotics in the treatment of schizophrenia: systematic overview and meta-regression analysis. *British Medical Journal, 321*(7273), 1371-1376.

Gilman, P. K. (2010, June). Bupropion, Bayesian logic and serotonin toxicity. *Journal of Medical Toxicology, 6*(2), 276-277.

Govtrack.us. (2003, December 93). S. 650 (108th): Pediatric Research Equity Act of 2003. Retrieved from https://www.govtrack.us/congress/bills/108/s650

Hassner Sharav, V. (2004, June 28). CDER FDA MedWatch Listserv- Effexor (venlafaxine) warnings added for neonatal effects and suicidality risk. Retrieved from http://www.ahrp.org/informail/04/06/29.php

Hayhow, B. D., Brockman, S., & Starkstein, S. E. (2014). Post-stroke depression. In T.A. Scheizer & R. L. Macdonald (Eds.) *The behavioral consequences of stroke* (227-240). New York, NY: Springer.

Healy, D. (2002). *The creation of psychopharmacology*. Cambridge, MA: Harvard University Press.

Hoyer, D., Hannon, J. P., & Martin, G. R. (2002, April). Molecular, pharmacological and functional diversity of 5-HT receptors. *Pharmacology, Biochemistry and Behavior, 71*(4), 533-554.

Janssen Pharmaceuticals, Inc. (2012, February 13). Topamax (topiramate) tablets. Retrieved from http://topamax.com

Johansson, B., Wentzel, A. P., Andréll, P., Odenstadt, J., Mannheimer, C., & Ronnbäck, L. (2013, December 30). Evaluation of dosage, safety and effects of methylphenidate on post-traumatic brain injury symptoms with a focus on mental fatigue and pain. *Brain Injury*, Epub ahead of print.

Kessler, R. C., Berglund, P., Borges, G., Nock, M., & Wang, P. S. (2005, May 25). Trends in suicide ideation, plans, gestures, and attempts in the United States, 1990-1992 to 2001-2003. *Journal of the American Medical Association, 293*(20), 2487-2495.

King, M. W. (12/13/2013). themedicalbiochemistrypage, LLC. Retrieved from http://www.themedicalbiochemistrypage.org.

Kudo, Y., & Kurihara, M. C. (1990). Clinical evaluation of diphenhydramine hydrochloride for the treatment of insomnia in psychiatric patients: a double-blind study. *Journal of Clinical Pharmacology, 30*(11), 1041-1048.

Kurwana, E. (2005, June). Gamma hydroxybutyrate (GHB). Retrieved from http://faculty.washington.edu/chudler/ghb.html.

Lallanilla, M. (Reporter). (February 3, 2004). Research Links Month of Birth to Disease [Video podcast]. ABC News. Retrieved from http://abcnews,go,com/Health/Story?id=118260.

Lieberman, J. (2003). History of the Use of Antidepressants in Primary Care. Primary Care Companion, *Journal of Clinical Psychiatry, 5*(suppl 7), 6-10.

Lieberman, J. A., Stroup, T. S., McEvoy, J. P., Swartz, M. S., Rosenheck, R. A., Perkins, D. O., Keefe, R. S., Davis, S. M., Davis, C. E., Lebowitz, B. D., Severe, J., & Hsiao, J. K. (2005). Effectiveness of antipsychotic drugs in patients with chronic schizophrenia. *New England Journal of Medicine, 353*(12), 1209-1223. doi: 10.1056/NEJMoa051688

Lieberman, L. A., & Higgins, D. E. (2009, February). A small-molecule screen identifies the antipsychotic drug pimozide as an inhibitor of Listeria monocytogenes infection. *Antimicrobial Agents and Chemotherapy, 53*(2), 756-764.

Medicines and Healthcare Products Regulatory Agency: MHRA cautions against cardiotoxicity of venlafaxine. (2004, December 6). Press Release- National Institute for Clinical Excellence, U.K. Retrieved from http://www.nice.org.uk/pdf/2004_50_launchdepressionanxietypdf.

139

Medicines and Healthcare Products Regulatory Agency: New advice issued on risperidone and olanzapine. (2005, September 5). Press Release- Committee for the Safety of Medicines, U.K. Retrieved from http://www.mhra.gov.uk/NewsCentre/Pressreleases/CON002047.

Magellan Health Services. (n.d.). A Patient's Handout for Citalopram/Escitalopram and the FDA Warning. Retrieved from http://www.magellanofaz/com/media/250425/citalopram%20bhr%.

Manfredi, R. L., & Kales, A. (1987, September). Clinical neuropharmacology of sleep disorders. *Seminars in Neurology, 7*(3), 286-295.

Mayberg, H. S., Silva, J. A., Brannan, S. K., Tekell, J. L., Mahurin, R. K., McGinnis, S., & Jerebek, P. A. (2002). The functional neuroanatomy of the placebo effect. *American Journal of Psychiatry, 159*(5), 728-737.

Merriman, D. (2012, March 27). Confirmation of Orphan Drug Designation for the use of fluoxetine for the treatment of autism. Retrieved from http://autismtherapeutics.com/at_new/wp-content/uploads/2012/12/AT-Press-Release-March-27-2012-ODD-Confirmation.pdf

Mesure, S. (2013). McKnight's Long-Term Care News & Assisted Living. Retrieved from http://www.mcknights.com/no-magic-pill-for-treating-sympstoms-of-alzheimers-study-finds/article/101465.

Moncrieff, J., Wessely, S., & Hardy, R. (2004). Active placebos versus antidepressants for depression. *Cochrane Database of Systematic Reviews* (1). doi: 10.1002/14651858.CD003012.pub.2

Muncie, Jr., H. L., Yasinian, Y., & Ogé, L. (2013, November). Outpatient management of alcohol withdrawal syndrome. *American Family Physician, 88*(9), 589-595.

Munhoz, R. P. (2004, September/October). Serotonin syndrome induced by a combination of bupropion and SSRIs. *Clinical Neuropharmacology, 27*(5), 219-222.

Myrick, H., Malcolm, R., & Brady, K. T. (1998, November). Gabapentin treatment of alcohol withdrawal. *The American Journal of Psychiatry, 155*(11), 1626.

Niedowski, E. (08/21/2004). Scientists link month of birth to diseases. *The Indianapolis Star*, NA.

Noh, Y., Kim, D. W., Chu, K., Jung, K. H., Moon, H. J., & Lee, S. K. (2013, January). Topiramate increases the risk of valproic acid-induced encephalopathy. *Epilepsia, 54*(1), e1-4. doi: 10.1111/j.1528-1167-2012-03532.x

Novartis Pharmaceuticals Corporation. (2013, January). Diagnosing and monitoring carcinoid syndrome. Retrieved from http://carcinoid.com/patient/understanding/carcinoid-syndrome-diagnosis.jsp?usetrack.filter_applied=true&Novald=4029462103691102715

O'Neil, M., Page, N., Adkins, W. N., & Eichelman, B. (1986, October 1). Tryptophan-trazodone treatment of aggressive behavior. *The Lancet, 2*(8511), 859-860.

Onishi, E., Biagioli, F., & Safranek, S. (2014, January 15). Methylphenidate for management of fatigue in the palliative care setting. *American Family Physician, 89*(2), 124-127.

Peters, R. L. (2013). Overview of Nervous System. Retrieved from http://www.otah0.wikispaces.com/09+Nervous+System.

Peveler, R., Kendrick, A., Buxton, M., Longworth, L., Baldwin, D., Moore, M., Chatwin, J., Goddard, J., Thornett, A., Smith, H., Campbell, M., & Thompson, C. (2004). A randomised controlled trial to compare the cost-effectiveness of tricyclic antidepressants, selective serotonin reuptake inhibitors, and lofepramine. *Health Technology Assessment, 9*(16), 1-134.

Poore, J. (2014, January 10). Serzone (nefazodone) synopsis. Retrieved from http://www.crazymeds.us/pmwiki/pmwiki.php/Meds.Serzone.

Poore, J. (2014, January 11). Topamax (topiramate) overview. Retrieved from http://www.crazymeds.us/pmwiki/pmwiki.php/Meds.Topamax.

Preskorn, S. H. (1999, November). Two in one: the venlafaxine story. *Journal of Practical Psychiatry and Behavioral Health, 5*(6), 1-5.

Pringle, E. (2007, February 19). OpEdNews.com: Suicide risk of Neurontin kept hidden for years. Retrieved from http://www. opednews.com/articles/genera_evelyn_p_070219_suicide_risk_of_neur.htm

Rai, D., Lee, B. K., Dalman, C., Lewis, G., & Magnusson, C. (2013, April 19). Parental depression, maternal antidepressant use during pregnancy, and risk of autism spectrum disorders: population based case-control study. *British Medical Journal.* doi: 10-1136/bmj.f2059

Rao, J. S., Lee, H. J., Rapoport, S. I., & Brazinet, R. P. (2008, June). Mode of action of mood stabilizers: is the arachidonic cascade a common target? *Molecular Psychiatry, 13*(8), 585-596.

Riding, J., & Munro, A. (1975, July). Pimozide in the treatment of monosymptomatic hypochondriacal psychosis. *Acta Psychiatrica Scandinavica, 52*(1), 23-30.

Roy, D., Hoffman, P., Dudas, M., & Mendelowitz, A. (2013). Pharmacologic management of aggression in adults with intellectual disability. *Journal of Intellectual Disability- Diagnosis and Treatment, 1*(1), 28-43. doi: 10.6000/2292-2598.2013.01.01.5

RxList: The Internet Drug Index. Desoxyn. (2013, December 13). Retrieved from http://www.rxlist.com/desoxyn-drug.htm.

Sachs, O. W. (1999). *Awakenings.* New York, NY: Vantage Books.

Schröck, A., Han, Y., König, S., Auwärter, V., Schürch, S., & Weinmann, W. (2013, June). Pharmacokinetics of GHB and detection window in serum and urine after single uptake of a low dose of GBL- an experiment with two volunteers. *Drug Testing and Analysis.* doi: 10.1002/dta.1498

Shorter, E. (1997). *A history of psychiatry: From the era of the asylum to the age of Prozac.* New York, NY: John Wiley & Sons, Inc.

Simon, G. E., Cunningham, M. L., & Davis, R. L. (2002, December 1). Outcomes of prenatal antidepressant exposure. *The American Journal of Psychiatry, 159*(12), 2055-2061.

Sinclair, L. I., Christmas, D. M., Hood, S. D., Potokar, J. P., Robertson, A., Isaac, A., Srivastava, S., Nutt, D. J., & Davies, S. J. (2009). Antidepressant-induced jitteriness/anxiety syndrome: systematic review. The British Journal of Psychiatry: *The Journal of Mental Science, 194*(6), 483-490. doi: 10 .1192/bjp.107.048371

Smith, T. A. (2014). *Aromatherapy: A primer for health professionals. The essential guide to essential oils.* Martinsville, IN: Smith Rehabilitation Consultants, Inc.

Spar, M. D., & Munóz, G. E. (2014). *Integrative men's health.* New York, NY: Oxford University Press.

Spratto, G. R., & Woods, A. L. (2013). *2013 Delmar healthcare drug handbook.* Clifton Park, NY: Delmar.

StopBadTherapy.com. (10/30/2013). Stop Bad Therapy. Retrieved from http://www.StopBadTherapy.com.

Surges, R., Volynski, K., & Walker, M. (2008). Is levetiracetam different from other antiepileptic drugs? Levetiracetam and its cellular mechanism of action in epilepsy revisited. *Therapeutic Advances in Neurological Disorders, 1*(1): 13-24.

The MIT Press: Cognition, Brain, & Behavior. Life and Mind. (2003). Retrieved from http://www.mitpress.mit.edu/books/new-phrenology.

Thorpe, E. L., Pizon, A. F., Lynch, M. J., & Boyer, J. (2010, June). Bupropion induced serotonin syndrome: a case report. *Journal of Medical Toxicology, 6*(2), 168-171.

U.S. Department of Health & Human Services, U.S. Food and Drug Administration. (2011, October 20). FDA drug safety communication: Serious CNS reactions possible when methylene blue is given to patient taking certain psychiatric medications. Retrieved from http://www.fda.gov/Drugs/DrugSafety/ucm263190.htm.

U.S. Department of Health & Human Services. U.S. Food and Drug Administration. (2012, March 28). FDA Drug Safety Communication: Revised recommendations for Celexa (citalopram hydrobromide) related to a potential risk of abnormal heart rhythms with high doses. Retrieved from http://www.fda.gov/Drugs/DrugSafety/ucm297391.htm.

U.S. Department of Health & Human Services. U.S. Food and Drug Administration. (2013, June 18). Zyprexa Relprevv (olanzapine pamoate): Drug Safety Communication- FDA investing two deaths following injection. Retrieved from http://www.fda.gov/Safety/MedWatch/SafetyInformation/SafetyAlertsforHumanMedicalProducts/ucm 356701.htm.

U.S. Food and Drug Administration: News and Events. FDA News Release. (2004, October 15). FDA launches a multi-pronged strategy to strengthen safeguards for children treated with antidepressant medications. Retrieved from http://www.fda.gov/NewsEvents/Newsroom/PressAnnouncements/2004/ucm108363.htm

U.S. Food and Drug Administration. (2011, March 4). News & Events, FDA News Release. For immediate release. FDA: Risk of oral birth defects in children born to mothers taking topiramate. Retrieved from http://www.fda.gov/NewsEvents/Newsroom/PressAnnouncements/ucmn245594.htm.

USA Today. Health and Behavior. The Associated Press. (2004, October 15). FDA orders warnings on antidepressants used by kids. Retrieved from http://www.ustoday30.ustoday.com/news/health/2004-10-15-drug-kids_x.htm.

USA Today. (01/20/2003). Health and Behavior. Retrieved from http://www.usatoday30usetoday.com/news/health/2003-01-20-children-drugs-x.htm.

U.S. Food and Drug Administration. (2006). Drug Safety and Risk Management Advisory Committee Meeting February 9 and 10, 2006. Retrieved from http://www.fda.gov/ohrms/dockets/ac/06/briefing/2006-4202_00_toc.htm.

U.S. Food and Drug Administration. (2013, December 2). Orphan Drug Designations and Approvals List as of 12-02-2013. Governs January 2014-March 2014. Retrieved from http://www.hrsa.gov/opa/programrequirements/orphandrugexlusion/orphandruglist.pdf.

United States National Library of Medicine: National Institute of Diabetes and Digestive and Kidney Diseases. (2013, November 5). LiverTox: Drug Record- Temazepam. Retrieved from http://www.livertox.nih.gov/Temazepam.htm.

Uttal, W. (2003). *The new phrenology- The limits of localizing cognitive processes in the brain.* Cambridge, MA: MIT Press.

van Vloten, W. A. (2003, March). Pimozide: Use in dermatology. *Dermatology Online Journal, 9*(2), 3.

von Wolff, A., Hölzel, L. P., Westphal, A., Härter, M., & Kriston, L. (2013, January). Selective serotonin reuptake inhibitors and tricyclic antidepressants in the acute treatment of chronic depression and dysthymia: A systematic review and meta-analysis. *Journal of Affective Disorders, 144*(1-2), 7-15.

Weiden, P. J. (2007, January). EPS profiles: the atypical antipsychotics are not all the same. *Journal of Psychiatric Practice, 13*(1), 13-24.

Weiner, M. A., & Goss, K. (1989). *The Complete Book of Homeopathy.* Garden City, NY: Avery.

Whitaker, R. (2010). *Anatomy of an epidemic: Magic bullets, psychiatric drugs, and the astonishing rise of mental illness in America.* New York, NY: Random House.

Wikipedia. (2013, August 12). Entorhinal cortex. Retrieved from http://www.en.wikipedia.org/wiki/Entorhinal_cortex.

Woolley, D. W. (1962). *The biochemical bases of psychosis or the serotonin hypothesis about mental diseases*. New York, NY: John Wiley and Sons, Inc.

155

Made in the USA
Lexington, KY
26 November 2017